DETOX

The PROCESS of CLEANSING and RESTORATION

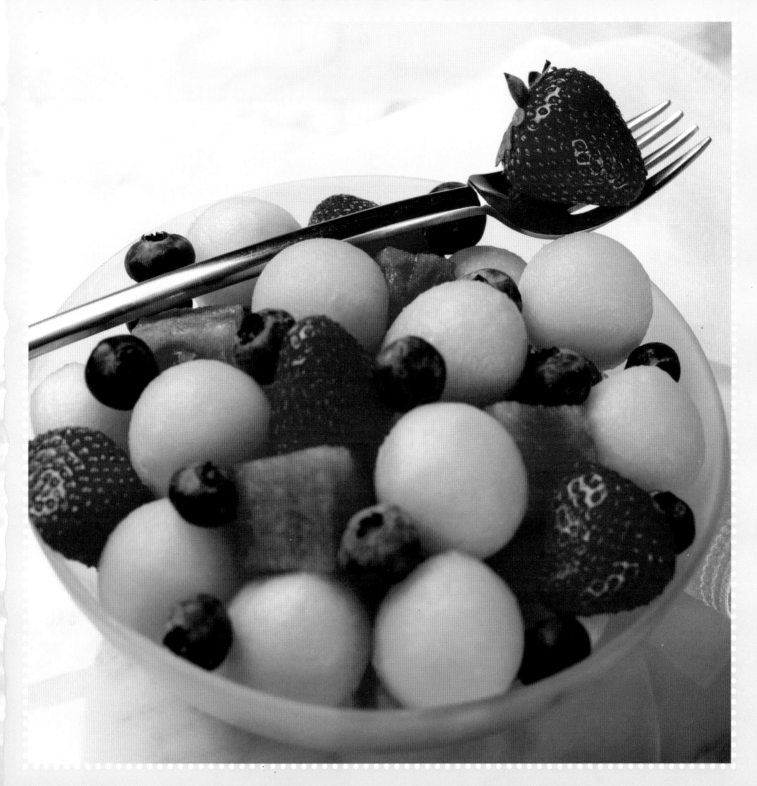

This is a Parragon Book

First published in 2004

Parragon

Queen Street House

4 Queen Street

Bath BA1 1HE, UK

ISBN: 1-40544-313-8

Printed in China

Produced by the Bridgewater Book Company Ltd

Photographer: Calvey Taylor-Haw

Note

As a precautionary measure, the publishers advise that anyone
intending to follow the programmes outlined in this book should
first consult a qualified medical practitioner.

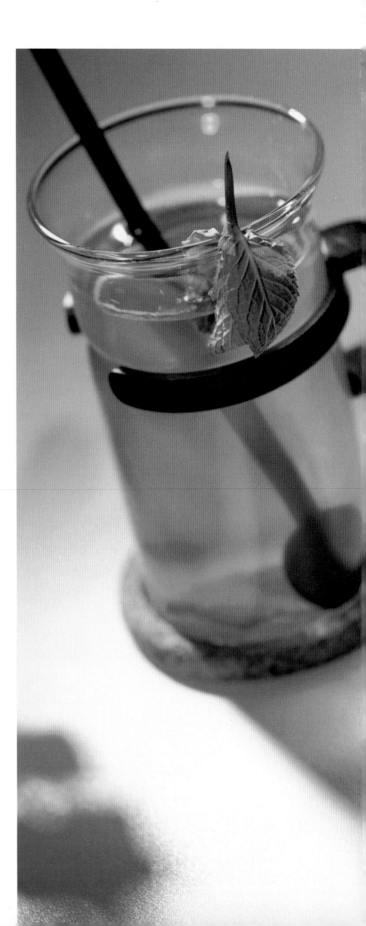

CONTENTS

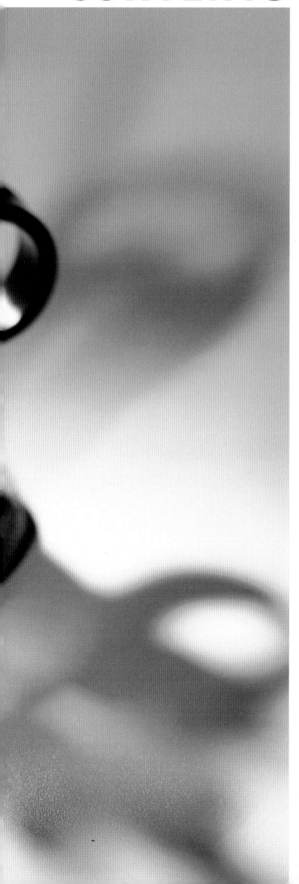

what is detoxing?

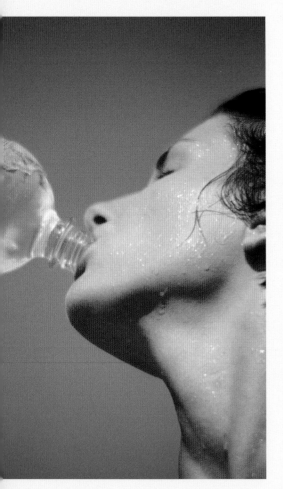

Detoxing is just another word for cleansing. The aims of a detox programme are to increase the efficiency of the digestive system and to stimulate the other parts of the body that are responsible for cleansing and elimination. Detoxing also works to improve underlying health so you are less prone to infection. Used sensibly and occasionally, detox regimes are invaluable in promoting and sustaining good health.

Ways of detoxing

Detoxing is a relative term. Anything that supports elimination will help you detox. Doing no more than drinking a couple of litres of water a day will help you flush out toxins. Eating more fresh fruit and vegetables – high water-content, cleansing foods – and fewer meat and dairy products will reduce congestion and increase elimination. However, it is important not to go to extremes – fasting, frequent enemas, use of diuretics and excessive exercise hold the danger of making you lose essential nutrients.

In this book, detoxing involves reducing the intake of toxins and improving their elimination through diet and body therapies such as spa treatments and skin brushing. You should also try to avoid chemicals, refined foods, sugar, caffeine, alcohol, tobacco and many drugs to reduce the toxic load.

The most important way of strengthening your body's natural defences and combating the daily onslaught of toxins is to improve your diet. Food can provide a rich source of antioxidants and plant chemicals, which improve the way your body eliminates waste products and increase your body's ability to remove pollutants.

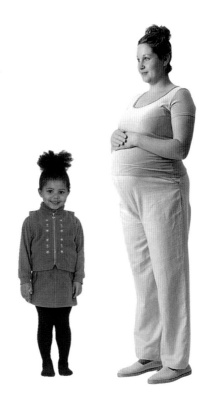

Your body is designed to cope with toxins, and neutralizes, transforms or eliminates them. The liver is the main organ of detoxification, transforming toxins into harmless agents so that they can then be eliminated. The kidneys filter out waste products from your blood into your urine. Your intestines propel potential toxins and indigestible material from food into the bowel for excretion. The lungs expel gases such as carbon dioxide which are produced in the cells and filter out poisonous gases you breathe in. The skin eliminates toxins via sweat and sebum (skin oil) and by shedding dead skin cells. The lymphatic system carries waste products that are too large to enter the bloodstream to the lymph nodes for processing. They are then returned to the liver via the bloodstream for detoxification.

Healing crises

As detoxification takes effect your health should improve steadily, possibly with temporary relapses known as healing crises. Minor ailments such as colds, fevers and skin spots should be seen in a positive light because they are signs that the body is trying to throw off an accumulation of toxins. So, don't be surprised if your skin becomes dull or spotty at the beginning of a detox programme – it will soon clear.

Who shouldn't detox

Children under the age of 18, pregnant or breastfeeding women, those who are ill or recovering from illness, and those over the age of 65 should not detox. If you have a medical condition or are taking medication, you must seek medical advice before detoxing as it may not be suitable for you.

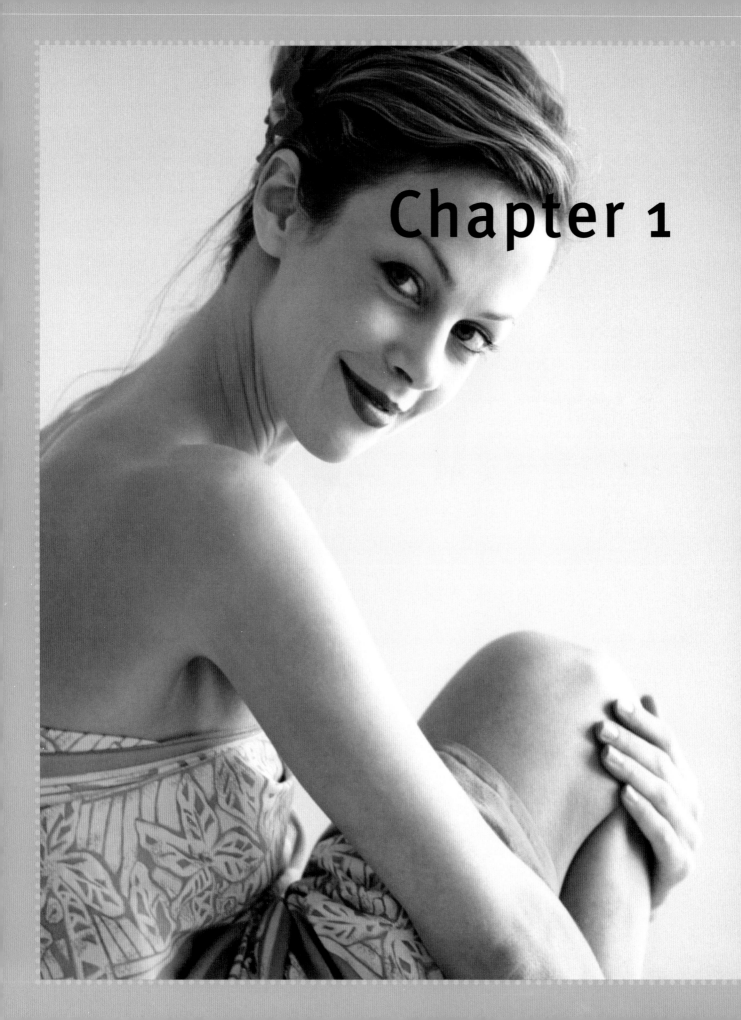

Chapter 1

ESSENTIAL
DETOX

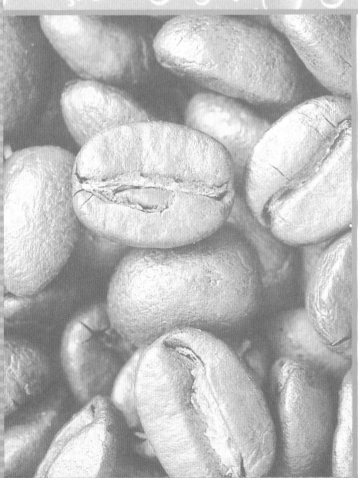

toxic overload

Stressful situations trigger your
body's fight-or-flight response, a
primitive biochemical reaction that
puts your body on red alert. If stress
then continues, physical and mental
health can be undermined as the
stress hormones adrenaline and
cortisol disrupt the functioning of the
immune and circulatory systems.
Thus your body becomes less
efficient at eliminating toxins, and
your toxic load increases.

A toxin is any substance that causes irritating or harmful effects in your body. We acquire toxins from our environment by breathing them in, by ingesting them or through physical contact. Every day we are exposed to new and stronger chemicals, air and water pollution, and radiation. We use more drugs, eat more sugar and refined foods, and turn to damaging props such as alcohol and tobacco to help us deal with rising stress levels. Internally, our bodies produce toxins through normal everyday functions. Biochemical, cellular and bodily activities generate substances that also need to be eliminated. Other factors such as lack of sleep, exercise or fresh air, and even negative attitudes, are thought to allow waste products and toxins to build up in the body and upset its self-regulation.

If your body is working well, with a good immune system and eliminative functions, you can deal with your everyday exposure to toxins. However, if you are taking in more toxins than you can eliminate, your body will reach a state of toxicity. If your digestive system is not functioning properly there may also be an overgrowth of destructive bacteria that encourage even more toxins to proliferate. A sluggish liver, blocked skin pores and congested lungs all add to increased toxicity.

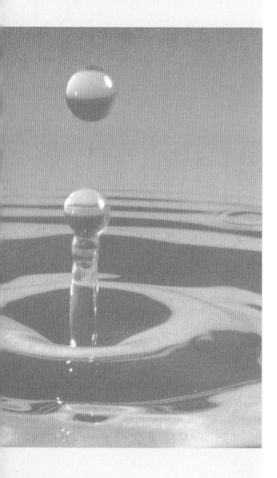

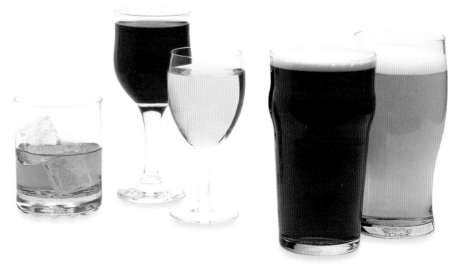

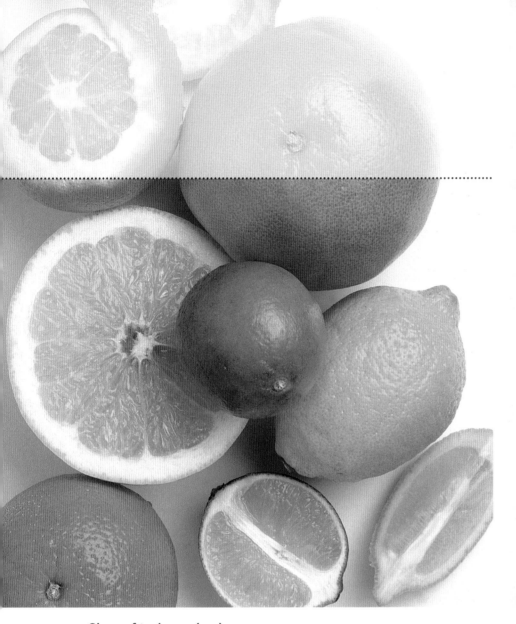

Free radicals are molecules made in all combustion processes, including frying and barbecuing food and smoking; they are also produced by the body as a natural by-product of metabolism. In small amounts they can fight invading bacteria and viruses; in large amounts they are thought to damage body cells, speeding up the ageing process, contributing to a range of illnesses and causing cholesterol to clog up the arteries. Free radicals are constantly being made and broken down. They can be neutralized by antioxidants in food, which seek them out and deactivate them. The main antioxidant nutrients are vitamins A, C and E, and the minerals selenium, zinc, manganese and copper. Bioflavonoids – chemical compounds found mainly in citrus fruits – are also extremely effective at ridding the body of any harmful free radicals.

Signs of toxic overload

Dry, blotchy, spotty skin, headaches, fungal infections, lack of energy, joint pain, allergies, wind, bloating, constipation or generally feeling under the weather may all be indications that your body has more toxins than it can handle, and that you would benefit from giving your system a good clean-out. Many of these symptoms may be linked to food intolerance, whereby it is thought that over time your body fails to digest certain foods properly. Food cravings or headaches after withdrawing a food from your diet may be signs that you are intolerant to a particular food, the most common culprits being wheat, cow's milk products, citrus fruits, soya, coffee, tea and other caffeinated drinks, and peanuts.

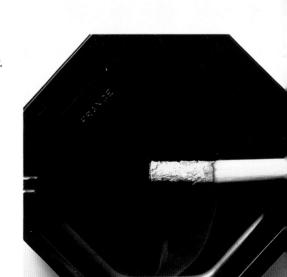

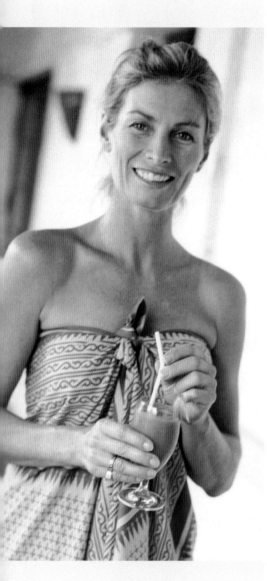

the benefits
of detox

Detoxing will improve your appearance, regulate your sleep patterns and boost your emotional well-being. It will increase your vitality and your underlying health and may also help you lose weight.

Improved appearance

One of the key benefits of detoxing is just how much better you will look. Apart from reducing bloating, streamlining your body and toning your muscles through the combination of diet and body therapies, your skin will be transformed. Expect your skin to look softer and better hydrated, your complexion to be clearer and the condition of your hair and nails to improve significantly. There should be less puffiness under your eyes and the eyes themselves should be clearer and brighter. You'll even find your teeth are brighter as you avoid discolouring tannins present in tea, coffee and red wine.

Better health

Detoxing improves the health of your immune system by increasing the amount of antioxidant nutrients that are key to fighting infection and disease. As a result you'll suffer from fewer colds and minor illnesses. If you've been suffering from a food intolerance without knowing it, you may even find that allergic disorders such as hayfever and eczema, as well as stomach cramps, diarrhoea and headaches, disappear once the offending item has been removed from your diet.

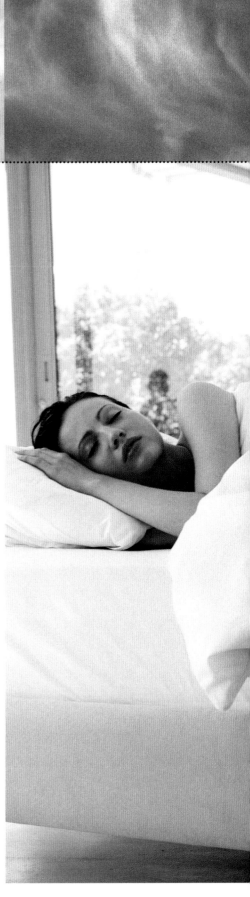

Restful sleep

Detoxing will help you sleep better because you will be eliminating so many harmful substances that have been keeping you awake. Many people use alcohol as a sedative, but in fact it is a stimulant in the same way as caffeine and tobacco, and will wake you up in the middle of the night. Regular exercise will also promote deeper sleep, but avoid anything too strenuous in the hours before bedtime. The relaxation therapies you will encounter in this book are also useful in helping you get a restful night.

Improved mood and inner harmony

Ridding your mind of negative thoughts will improve your outlook and do wonders for your state of health. Research has shown that optimism and happiness are strongly linked to good health, increased well-being and your body's potential to heal itself. Healthy eating will stabilize your blood sugar levels, which in turn will prevent your moods from fluctuating, helping you to feel more relaxed and better able to deal with stress. Meditation and visualization techniques will enable you to detoxify your mind.

Weight loss

Anyone who regularly eats thousands of calories of fatty, sugary and nutritionally unsound food a day will lose weight if they follow this detox programme. However, weight loss is only an added bonus, not the main aim. Don't be tempted to weigh yourself while detoxing because if you find you haven't lost any weight you might not feel motivated to carry on.

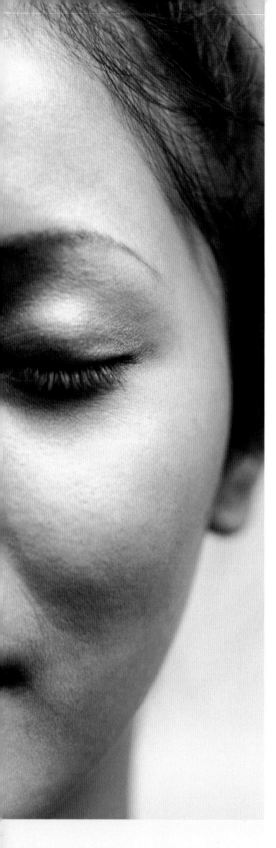

aims of detox

The aims of a detox programme are to reduce the workload of the digestive system, allowing it to perform more efficiently, and to stimulate the parts of your body that are responsible for cleansing and elimination. Successful detoxing depends for the main part on what you eat and drink, but it can be complemented by body therapies to speed up the elimination of toxins, and mind therapies to help you relax and reduce stress levels. The intention is to coax your mind and body to rid itself of waste, replacing it with revitalizing and nurturing foods and thoughts.

The food detox programme improves the digestive system and immunity; reduces your exposure to toxins; and, finally, increases the actions of the liver and kidneys, the main organs of detoxification. It will provide you with everything you need for a full internal spring clean. However, to get the most out of detoxing you need to look after your mind as well as your body. Well-being depends on maintaining a balance between your emotional, mental, spiritual and physical health, and if this balance is upset it disrupts your body's harmony and leads to ill health. The body and mind detox programme contains simple yet effective techniques that will help you to look after your body and encourage a positive state of mind to promote all-round well-being and good health.

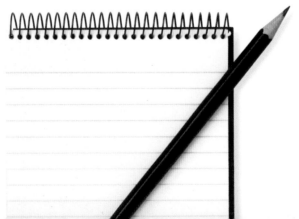

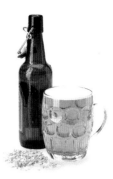

ASSESS YOUR TOXIC LOAD

Answer the following questions as truthfully as you can. Score 1 point for every yes, 0 for no. Unless you score 5 points or less, you should break yourself in gently by following the Countdown to Detox programme on pages 16–17 to prevent headaches and side effects that come from detoxing too quickly. There is no right or wrong score here, but you should keep your score so that you can measure your progress after completing the detox programme.

1. Do you feel tired when you wake up in the morning even though you've had enough sleep?
2. Do you drink more than 3 cups of coffee, tea or caffeinated fizzy drinks such as cola a day?
3. Do you suffer from skin rashes, spots around the mouth or eczema?
4. Do you suffer from bloating after meals?
5. Do you have an alcoholic drink most days?
6. Do you smoke or live with smokers?
7. Do you live or work in a city?
8. Do you rarely eat fresh fruit or vegetables?
9. Do you eat red meat more than twice a week?
10. Do you eat fried food and junk foods?
11. Do you suffer from constant colds, hay fever or allergies?
12. Do you have mood swings?
13. Do you crave certain foods such as sweets and bread?
14. Do you skip meals, especially breakfast?
15. Do you put on weight easily?
16. Do you find it difficult to concentrate?
17. Do you often have irregular bowel movements (i.e. constipation or diarrhoea)?
18. Do your joints or muscles sometimes ache?
19. Do you feel tired and lethargic most of the time?
20. Do you suffer from fungal infections such as thrush, athlete's foot or ringworm?

GO ORGANIC?

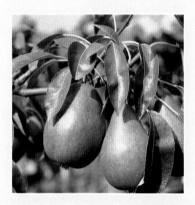

Organic foods are not essential when detoxing – the very fact that you are increasing the amount of fruit and vegetables you consume will make a significant difference to how you look and feel. Furthermore, despite some recent food scares, the non-organic food that you can buy in the supermarket is stringently tested and carefully stored and transported and so should be safer than ever before.

However, organic foods are an attractive alternative for the consumer, offering food that will have been produced with minimal use of pesticides and other chemicals, and which adheres to standards set down by European law.

Most supermarkets stock organic produce, or you can have supplies delivered to you from organic wholesalers. The trick is to buy little and often, because organic food will go off more quickly.

To ensure that your detox programme goes as smoothly as possible, it is useful to gather together various items before you start. These include kitchen items to help you prepare meals more easily, and bathroom accessories to facilitate your body detox routine.

For the kitchen

- Airtight storage containers such as Tupperware® or Kilner® jars in which to keep dried foods
- Metal or bamboo steamer – the type you put over or in a pan of water to steam vegetables. This is an excellent way of cooking vegetables while retaining maximum flavour and nutrients
- Food processor to reduce chopping times
- Salad spinner to shake excess water off lettuce
- Juicer – a luxury item but worth it if it helps you consume more fresh fruit and vegetables

For the bathroom

- Skin brush with natural bristles, which should be firm but not too stiff or they may irritate your skin
- Loofah or flannel mitt (towelling or natural fibre)
- Exfoliating Scrub (see recipe page 65) or salt
- Your favourite essential oil, added to a suitable carrier oil (see page 71)

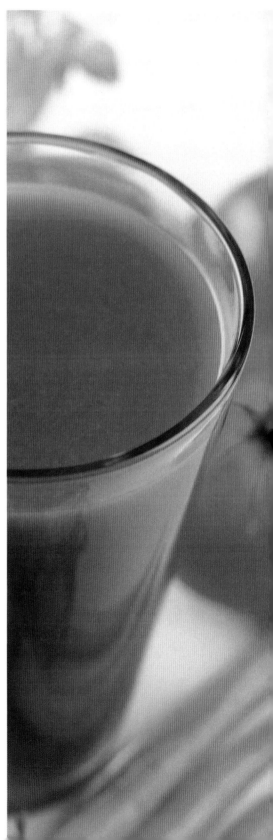

Detoxing your kitchen

A key step to successful detoxing is to clear your kitchen of all the fatty, sugar-laden comfort foods that you reach for in times of emotional crises so that, if you do go through a wobbly patch, there won't be anything bad in the cupboard for you to eat. Set aside a day to go through your cupboards and throw out all the processed and refined foods you find there. Then restock your kitchen with nutritionally sound food, using the shopping list on pages 24–25 for guidance. Where possible, choose locally grown fruits and vegetables – these retain more nutrients and cause less environmental damage because they don't have to be flown across the world to reach you.

Once you have the right ingredients, make a sustained effort to be more creative in the kitchen. Try out new recipes and new foods and discover just how delicious and satisfying your meals can be.

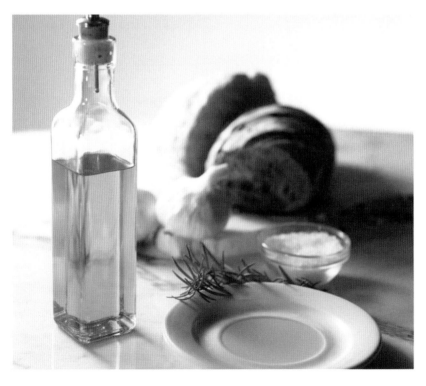

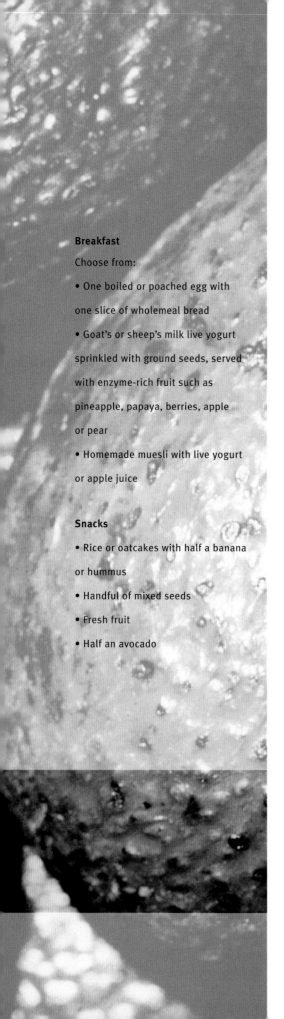

Breakfast

Choose from:

• One boiled or poached egg with one slice of wholemeal bread

• Goat's or sheep's milk live yogurt sprinkled with ground seeds, served with enzyme-rich fruit such as pineapple, papaya, berries, apple or pear

• Homemade muesli with live yogurt or apple juice

Snacks

• Rice or oatcakes with half a banana or hummus

• Handful of mixed seeds

• Fresh fruit

• Half an avocado

countdown
to detox

If you are nutritionally deficient or suffering from stress and fatigue, you must implement some preliminary changes before starting to detox. The aim is to improve the health of your digestive system and build up your immunity. If you follow this programme for two weeks it will ease you into detoxing and reduce the risk of experiencing unpleasant side effects such as headaches and tiredness.

Wean yourself off alcohol

Reduce your alcohol intake so that by the end of the fortnight it is down to little or nothing. This will reduce the liver's workload, the main organ of detoxification.

Start exercising

Take a walk at lunchtime, build up the amount of time you spend doing it and step up the pace.

Keep a food diary

Note down everything you eat and drink, the times, the approximate quantities and relevant details such as whether or not the products are organic. This will help you towards eating more healthily.

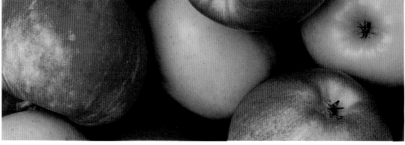

Cut down on caffeine

Reduce your consumption of tea, coffee and fizzy drinks. Do this by gradually replacing them over the course of a fortnight with herbal teas, fruit and vegetable juices and water. If you drink a lot of caffeinated drinks and give them up overnight, you will experience unpleasant side effects such as headaches, sleeplessness and irritability.

Drink more water

Increase your intake of fluids to at least 1.5 litres (3 pints) a day.

Eat more fruit and vegetables

Increase the amount of fruit and vegetables in your diet so that by the end of the fortnight you are consuming at least three portions of each every day. Apples, pears, pineapple and berry fruits are good choices at this stage and will speed up the passage of food through the intestines. Avoid citrus fruits for now because they are potent cleansers. Sweet potatoes, squashes and root vegetables are gentle on the digestive system.

Cut down on carbohydrates

Reduce your consumption of bread and pasta to one portion a day (one slice of bread or one heaped tablespoon of cooked pasta).

Lunch and dinner

Choose from the following and accompany with a green salad and Basic Salad Dressing (see page 58):

- Oily fish or organic poultry
- Vegetarian option based around tofu, pulses, grains such as rice, millet or quinoa, with a handful of nuts or seeds
- Grains with stir-fried or steamed vegetables. Choose a selection of brightly coloured vegetables such as tomatoes, peppers, broccoli and carrots, which are all rich in antioxidants and plant nutrients
- Baked potato (no more than three times a week)

For puddings, choose enzyme-rich berries, papaya or pineapple with live yogurt; in winter try baked apple or pear.

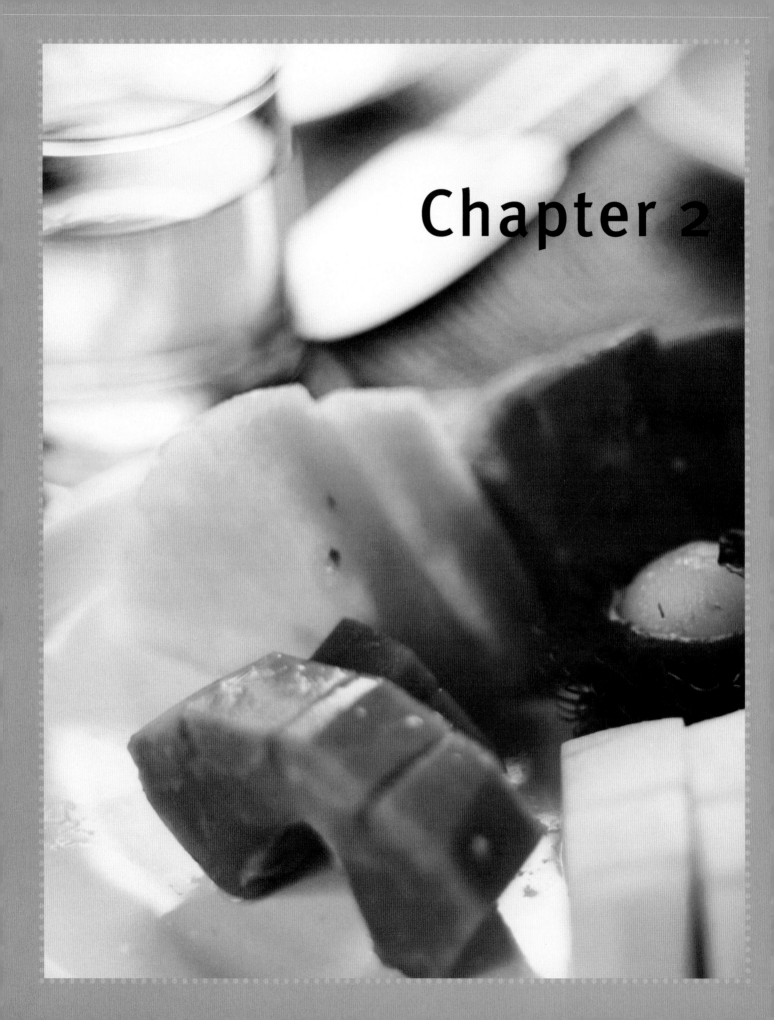

Chapter 2

FOOD DETOX

Don't be daunted at the prospect of giving up certain familiar foods – there is a wide range of delicious and nutritious alternatives.

Wheat products

Wheat-free bread; pasta made from corn, millet, rice or quinoa; buckwheat or rice noodles; brown rice, quinoa, millet; muesli made from oat, rye or millet flakes and oat porridge; corn tortillas.

Dairy products

Replace cow's milk with almond, oat, goat's or sheep's milk, or soya milk products. Instead of butter, use hummus, cashew nut or almond butter, or tahini.

Coffee and tea

Drink herbal teas, water, green tea, Rooibosch tea, chicory or dandelion root coffee (check that this does not contain lactose) and freshly squeezed fruit and vegetable juices instead.

Salt and sugar

Replace salt with seaweed and herbal salt substitutes. Use fresh herbs and spices to give bland foods flavour. Replace sugar with pure organic honey or maple syrup.

what to avoid

Successful detoxing depends for the most part on what you choose to eat and drink. This section tells you what foods you should choose or avoid while detoxing, what supplements you can take, and how to prepare your food to ensure you get the maximum amount of nutrients from it.

The foods to avoid when detoxing are those that are widely recognized as best limited or avoided in your diet in order to maintain good health, such as alcohol, caffeine, red meat and junk foods.

Cow's milk products

Milk increases the production of mucus in the body so it is not beneficial when detoxing. It is also thought that many people lack sufficient quantities of the enzyme lactase, which is needed to digest lactose (the main sugar in milk) and therefore cannot properly digest dairy products.

Tea, coffee, chocolate & other caffeinated drinks

Caffeine is a diuretic and leads to dehydration. As a stimulant it puts your body under stress and deprives it of essential nutrients. It also prevents your body from absorbing vitamins and minerals.

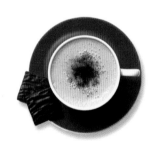

Alcohol

You should definitely give up alcohol while detoxifying. As well as containing sugar, alcohol is broken down into a toxin in your body, and the production of harmful free radicals is increased when it is being metabolized. Alcohol damages the liver, muscles and brain, and depletes your body of essential vitamins and minerals.

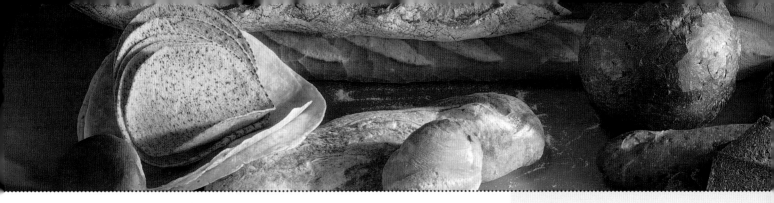

Wheat

Wheat bran can irritate the colon. Wheat protein (gluten) is difficult to
digest, and may cause bloating, constipation and/or diarrhoea. Gluten is
also present in oats, barley and rye, but there is significantly less in these
three grains. Many people are intolerant of wheat but find they can
consume other grains without problems. However, if you have coeliac
disease you will need to avoid all sources of gluten permanently.

Convenience foods, fatty and/or fried foods
and products containing sugar

These include ready meals, biscuits, cakes and spreads. Squashes and
cordials also contain sugar. Diet versions are not suitable alternatives
because of the amount of additives they contain. Choose fresh or dried
fruits and wholefood products instead, and drink water or fruit juices.

Meat

Meat creates extra work for your digestive system and in the case of red
meat contains a lot of harmful saturated fat. Eat small quantities of good
quality, organic protein instead to give your body the amino acids it needs.
Eggs, oily fish (from unpolluted waters) and soya are good choices.

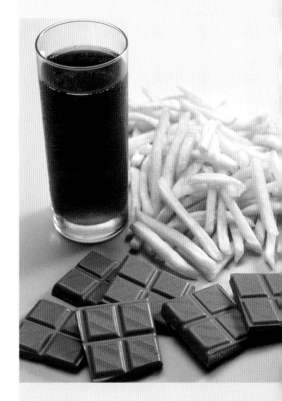

Salt and sugar

Your body needs a great deal of fluid to metabolize foods that are high in
refined sugar, so if you eat a lot of these foods your body will retain a lot
of water as well. Sugar disrupts blood glucose (sugar) levels. Salt prevents
fluid from being removed from the body.

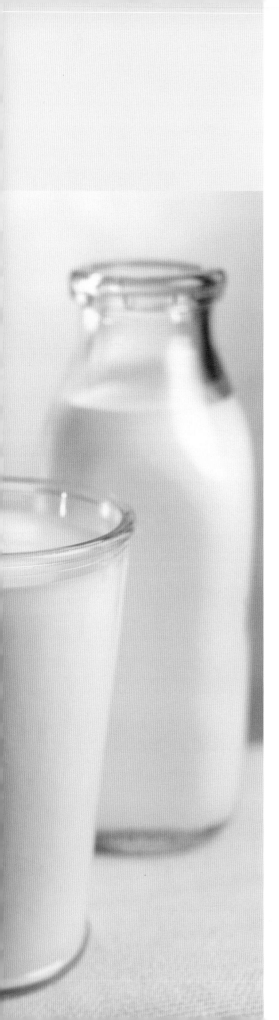

foods to choose

One of the key ways to detox is to keep the body in an alkaline state. The body's acid–alkaline balance adjusts throughout the day depending on the types of food we eat. Grains and proteins leave an acidic residue when metabolized; fruit and vegetables leave an alkaline residue. Protein and grains are essential for our overall health and well-being but if you balance their intake with large amounts of fruit and vegetables your body is more likely to remain alkaline. Choose organic food and eat fruit and vegetables raw whenever possible to make sure you obtain the maximum amount of nutrients.

The importance of fluids

Drinking plenty of fluids – at least 1.5 litres (3 pints) a day – is essential for good health. It will help avoid fluid retention and keep your body's waste disposal system – the liver, kidneys, lungs, digestive system, lymphatic system and skin – functioning efficiently. Water flushes out toxic materials, reduces bloating, helps keep your skin clear and is essential for a successful detox.

Drink fluids throughout the day, reducing the intake in the hours leading up to bedtime so that you do not have to get up in the night. Drinking with meals dilutes the digestive enzymes, so try to avoid drinking just before or up to an hour after meals. Herbal teas are excellent alternatives to water, and green tea and Rooibosch tea are rich in antioxidants. Freshly squeezed fruit and vegetable juices are loaded with nutrients, antioxidants and enzymes and help to keep your system alkaline, but they need to be drunk immediately as the nutrients are destroyed on exposure to air.

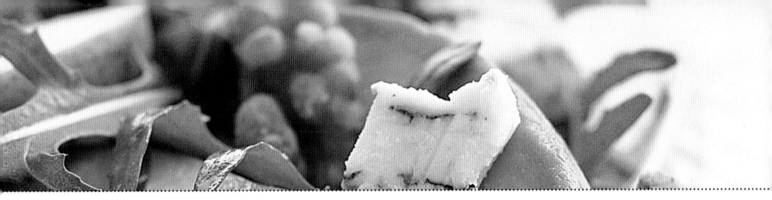

DETOX SUPERFOODS

Consume the following as often as you can.

Apple •• Helps excrete heavy metals and cholesterol and is cleansing for the liver and kidneys

Asparagus •• Superb detox food because of its diuretic effect; helps maintain healing bacteria in the intestines

Broccoli •• Like sprouts and cabbage, increases levels of glutathione, a key antioxidant that helps the liver expel toxins

Carrot •• Packed with beta-carotene, a powerful antioxidant; antibacterial and antifungal

Cranberry •• Antioxidant-rich; destroys harmful bacteria in the kidneys, bladder and urinary tract

Fennel •• Has a strong diuretic action and helps the body eliminate fats

Garlic •• Powerful antioxidant that is also excellent at eliminating toxic micro-organisms

Ginger •• Relieves abdominal bloating, nausea and diarrhoea. Helps to stimulate digestive enzymes, aiding efficient digestion

Globe artichoke •• Purifies and protects the liver and has a diuretic effect on the kidneys

Lemon •• Stimulates the release of enzymes – an essential part of the liver's detoxification process

Olive oil •• Antioxidant; prevents cholesterol from being transformed into a harmful free radical

Onion •• Rich in the antioxidant quercetin, which protects against free radical damage; onion enhances the activity of healthy intestinal flora and is antiviral

Parsley •• Diuretic and helps kidneys to flush out toxins; contains phytonutrients that support the liver and is rich in antioxidants

Quinoa •• Easily digested cleansing grain that is a good source of protein, vitamins and minerals

Rice •• Brown rice in particular cleans the intestines as it passes through and prevents constipation; anti-allergenic and helps stabilize blood-sugar levels

Salad leaf •• Superb antioxidant and cleanser of the digestive tract

Seaweed •• Strong antioxidant; helps alkalinize the blood and strengthens the digestive tract

Tomato •• Rich source of the antioxidant lycopene, thought to prevent a variety of diseases

Watercress •• Purifies the blood and expels wastes from the body

Yogurt •• Live yogurt contains probiotics that reduce intestinal inflammation and fungal infections and eliminate bad bacteria that damage the gut wall

shopping list

Fruit

Apples	Lemons
Apricots	Limes
Avocados	Lychees
Bananas	Mangoes
Blackberries	Melons
Blackcurrants	Nectarines
Blueberries	Olives
Cherries	Papaya
Cranberries	Passion fruit
Currants	Peaches
Damsons	Pears
Dates	Pineapples
Figs	Plums
Gooseberries	Prunes
Grapefruit	Raisins
Grapes	Raspberries
Greengages	Rhubarb
Guavas	Strawberries
Kiwi fruit	Sultanas
	Watermelons

Here is an at-a-glance checklist containing all the foods and drinks you are permitted while detoxing. You are not expected to sample everything but do try to get a good variety. Buy seasonal produce for best value.

Vegetables

Artichokes	Leeks
Asparagus	Lettuces
Aubergines	Marrows
Beans (e.g.	Okra
French, broad,	Onions
runner)	Parsnips
Beetroot	Peas
Broccoli	Peppers
Brussels sprouts	Potatoes
Cabbages	Pumpkins
Carrots	Radishes
Cauliflowers	Rocket
Celeriac	Spring greens
Celery	Squash
Chicory	Swedes
Chinese leaf	Sweetcorn
Courgettes	Sweet potatoes
Cucumbers	Turnips
Fennel	Watercress
Garlic	Yams

Grains

Brown rice	Oats
Buckwheat	Quinoa
Millet	Wheat-free pasta

Pulses and beansprouts

Bean sprouts	Butter beans
(e.g. mung,	Chickpeas
alfalfa,	Haricot beans
chickpeas)	Lentils
Black-eyed beans	Red kidney beans

Nuts and seeds

Almonds	Pecan
Brazil	Pine
Cashew	Pumpkin
Chestnuts	Sesame
Flax (linseed)	Sunflower
Hazelnuts	Walnuts
Macadamia	

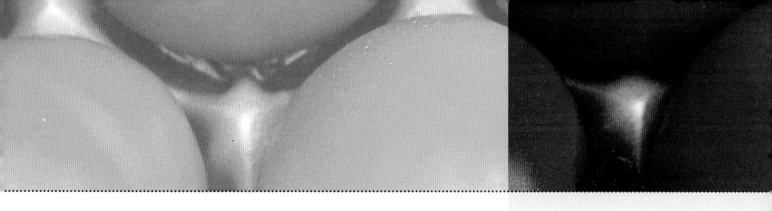

Herbs and spices

Basil	Marjoram
Cardamom pods	Mint
Cayenne pepper	Oregano
Chilli	Paprika
Chives	Parsley
Coriander	Pepper
Cumin	Rosemary
Dill	Tarragon
Fennel	Thyme
Ginger	Turmeric

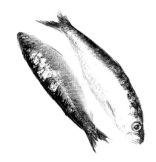

Fish

Anchovies	Pilchards
Cod	Plaice
Crab	Salmon
Haddock	Sardines
Halibut	Skate
Herring	Trout
Mackerel	Tuna

Drinks

Fruit juices	Mineral water
Green tea	Rooibosch tea
Herbal teas	Vegetable juices

Miscellaneous

Mustard (grain)	Seaweed
Oatcakes	Tahini
Quorn®	Tofu
Rice cakes	Wheat-free bread

Non-bovine dairy products

Almond milk	Sheep's cheese
Goat's cheese	Sheep's milk
Goat's milk	Sheep's yogurt
Goat's yogurt	Soya milk
Oat milk	Soya yogurt
Rice milk	

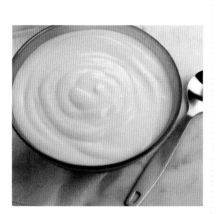

Oils and vinegars

Balsamic vinegar	Hazelnut oil
Cider vinegar	Lemon oil
Extra virgin olive oil	Sesame oil
	Sunflower oil
Grape seed oil	Walnut oil

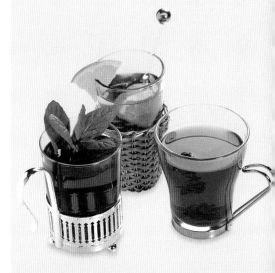

detox
supplements

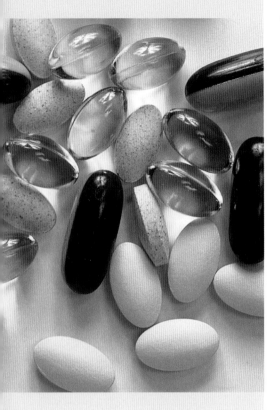

Supplements are usually taken as a nutritional safeguard against possible vitamin and mineral deficiencies caused by modern diets. When you are detoxing there are several supplements you can take that support the digestive processes and help nutrient absorption. You shouldn't need to take a specific antioxidant supplement – if you are eating a variety of fruit and vegetables you will be meeting your body's requirements. Too much vitamin C can cause diarrhoea and stomach upsets, while excessive amounts of vitamin A can be toxic. A general multivitamin/multimineral supplement, however, is normally fine, though you should seek advice from a qualified person before taking any supplements.

Unless otherwise stated on the packaging, supplements should be taken after food and washed down with water. Some can cause indigestion or make you feel sick if eaten on an empty stomach.

BLUE-GREEN ALGAE
These are a rich source of over 100 easily assimilated nutrients including antioxidants, vitamins, minerals, enzymes, essential fatty acids, amino acids and proteins. A number of blue-green algae are widely available in supplement form, for example aphanizomenon, chlorella and spirulina. Dosage: 500–1500 mg twice a day, best taken with food.

CO-ENZYME Q10
This is a substance needed by enzymes to help in energy production. Co-enzyme Q10 is particularly active in the liver, where it helps in the breakdown of toxins. This powerful antioxidant also helps to keep the heart healthy. Dosage: 10–100 mg daily, best taken with food.

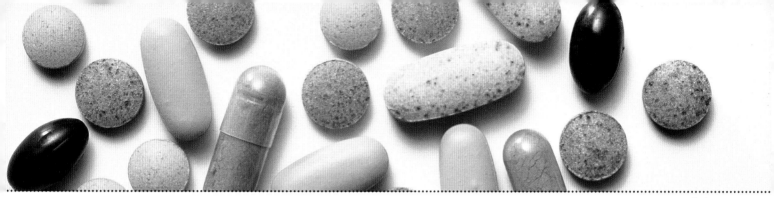

DANDELION

This increases the breakdown of dietary fats by stimulating the release of bile from the gallbladder. It is an extremely effective diuretic because of its high levels of potassium. Dosage: 500 mg twice a day.

KELP

These supplements are derived from seaweeds and contain vitamins, amino acids and minerals. Kelp is a particularly rich source of calcium, magnesium, potassium, iron and iodine. Iodine improves production of thyroid hormones, which boost metabolic rate and may therefore help weight loss. Dosage: depends on the supplement – take according to manufacturer's instructions. Note that some people are sensitive to iodine and taking kelp supplements can cause allergic reactions.

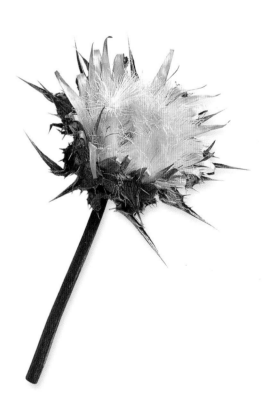

MILK THISTLE

The active compound in this antioxidant herb is silymarin, which helps repair the liver by encouraging the replacement of damaged liver cells with healthy ones. It also increases levels of glutathione, which helps remove alcohol, metals and pesticides from the body. Dosage: 120–160 mg three times a day.

PSYLLIUM HUSKS

These husks contain insoluble fibre, which loosens old matter in the bowel and increases the bulk of stools, and soluble fibre, which absorbs toxins in the bowel. Dosage: 1000–3000 mg one to three times a day with at least 500 ml water. Not to be taken with food.

Sprouts have a high vitamin and mineral content, and you can toss them into salads to make a nutritious dish. Aduki beans, alfalfa, chickpeas, mung beans and mustard cress are particularly easy to grow at home. Remove any split seeds and put about two tablespoonfuls into a tray, dish or jam jar, cover with tepid water and leave to soak overnight, covered with a piece of muslin. The following day, drain and rinse the seeds. Grains should be damp but not lying in water. Continue to drain and rinse with tepid water two or three times a day until they sprout. You can also buy beans ready sprouted from wholefood shops and some supermarkets. Keep them in the refrigerator, rinse before using and consume within three days of purchase.

preparing food

Shop little and often so that you have a constant supply of fresh fruit and vegetables, and store them in the dark. Prepared salads and chopped fruit and vegetables may seem convenient, but once they are chopped and exposed to light and oxygen they start to lose nutrients. Fruit and vegetables should not be washed or cut until you are ready to eat them. Leave the skins of fruit and vegetables on when possible because many essential nutrients are found just beneath the skin. However, if your vegetables are not organic, peel or throw away the outer leaves to reduce your exposure to pesticide residues.

COOKING

Try to cook your food as little as possible. Cooking alters the molecules in food and destroys many valuable nutrients and enzymes, and the longer you cook food the more nutrients it loses.

Steaming is the most effective way of cooking your vegetables. Boiling soups and stews is fine, however, because you consume the cooking liquid, which retains the nutrients.

If you stir-fry food it is cooked very briefly and, therefore, retains more nutrients. Use stock or water instead of oil because frying food in oil at high temperatures produces free radicals that destroy essential fatty acids in food. Onions and garlic, the basis of many savoury recipes, work well sautéed (pan-fried) in vegetable stock or water instead of butter or oil.

Use an oil and water spray
Make yourself an oil-and-water misting spray for when you need to grease a dish or lightly oil vegetables for grilling. Buy a plastic, spray atomizer

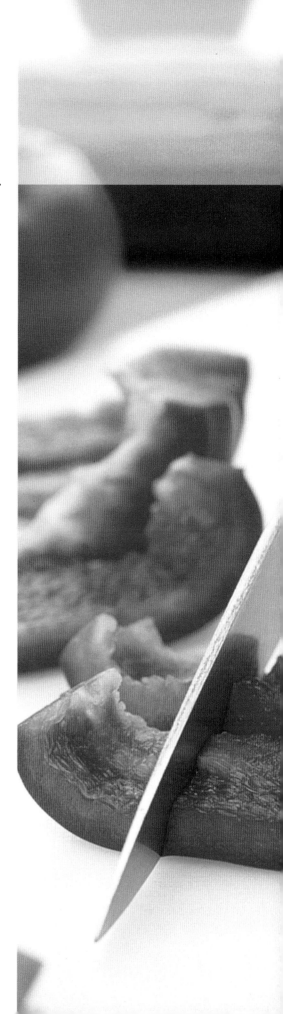

bottle and fill it with seven parts water and one part olive oil. Always shake the bottle first, then spray lightly. The water will evaporate in the cooking, leaving a bare minimum of oil.

Oil

Oils should be cold-pressed (cold pressing oils prevents damage to the essential fats caused by heat processing). Use extra virgin olive oil.

Pepper

Unless otherwise stated, always use freshly ground black pepper.

Nuts and seeds

These should be eaten unsalted. Lightly toast nuts and seeds by putting them in a hot oven for a few minutes or under the grill to bring out their nutty flavour. If the seeds are semi-sprouted, their nutritional value is increased.

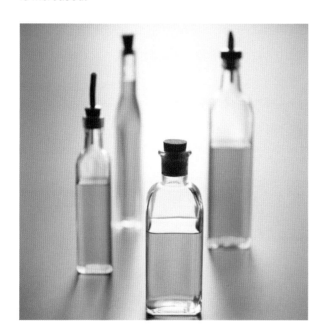

Here are some ideas for healthy snacks if you are feeling peckish between meals:

- Carrot and celery sticks with Hummus (see page 38)
- Small handful of nuts, seeds or raisins
- Piece of fresh fruit (e.g. apple, pear, slice of melon)
- Handful of grapes
- Portion of soya yogurt
- Glass of freshly squeezed fruit or vegetable juice
- Handful of olives

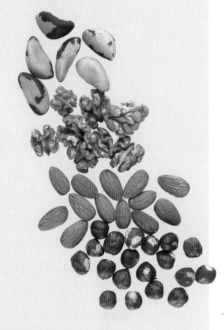

following the detox programme

The food detox programme covers a four-week period, with menu suggestions of what to eat while detoxing for every day of the week, from breakfast to dinner. The menus are designed to ensure you get the nutrients you need daily while building up your body's ability to flush out toxins. Recipes for the key dishes are given. If you don't like a particular ingredient or wish to create your own programme, you can swap meals around or substitute ingredients as long as your daily intake includes all the nutrition essentials listed here and your diet is full of variety. Missing out on a food category will make you feel sluggish because you won't be getting all your nutrients. In the long term, it is not good for health.

You can substitute different varieties of grains, fruits, vegetables, nuts and seeds according to preference, availability and cost. Soya yogurt is specified as it contains beneficial plant nutrients, but if you prefer, you can have goat's milk or ewe's milk yogurt. As this is not a weight-loss diet, quantities are not stated – just be sensible with high-fat foods such as nuts and avocados. In general you can eat as much salad, fruit and vegetables as you wish.

Daily nutrition essentials

- 1–2 portions of fat: e.g. seeds (see page 24), olive or seed oil, oily fish
- 2–3 portions of protein: choose vegetarian and fish sources such as eggs, soya products, lentils, beans, quinoa and oily fish rather than meat, to avoid the saturated fat
- 3 portions of fresh or dried fruit

- 3–4 portions of wholegrains: e.g. brown rice, millet, oats, corn and non-wheat pasta
- 5 portions of dark-green leafy and root vegetables
- At least 1.5 litres (3 pints) of liquid during the day, more if it is hot or you are exercising

  (Note: a portion is equivalent to a heaped tablespoon.)

When to eat

By making sure that you eat regularly you will help to keep your blood-sugar levels stable as well as helping to prevent binge-eating. Don't skip breakfast even if you're not feeling particularly hungry – breakfast kick-starts your metabolism and if you miss it you may feel tired and unable to concentrate. To give your body time to digest and absorb food prior to your next meal you should aim to have breakfast before 9 a.m., lunch before 2 p.m. and dinner before 7 p.m.

Daily detox essentials

- Drink a glass of hot water into which you have squeezed the juice of half a lemon first thing in the morning. This will help flush out your liver, the main organ of detoxification, and cleanse your palate
- Eat a clove of garlic in your food
- Eat a handful of unsulphured dried apricots
- Drink a cup of hot water with a teaspoon of fresh honey
- Eat a minimum of three meals a day

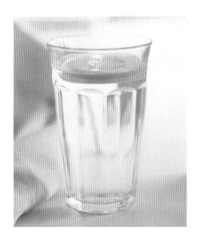

MEAL PLANNER

The following pages contain suggested menus that are carefully planned to build up your body's ability to flush out toxins. Have a piece of fruit to finish off a meal if you wish but avoid citrus fruits until week three because these are very powerful cleansers.

WEEK ONE

MONDAY

Breakfast	Fresh Fruit Muesli (see page 36)
Lunch	Tomato & Courgette Soup (see page 41) with wheat-free bread
Dinner	Baked potato with wild/organic grilled salmon, mackerel (substitute Hummus [see page 38] if vegetarian) and mixed leaf salad with Basic Salad Dressing (see page 58)

TUESDAY

Breakfast	½ melon filled with mixed berries (e.g. strawberries, raspberries, blackcurrants)
Lunch	Olive, Sun-dried Tomato & Lentil Pâté with Crudités (see page 39)
Dinner	Garden Paella (see page 52); Fresh Fruit Salad (see page 56)

WEDNESDAY

Breakfast	Boiled egg and wheat-free toast with honey
Lunch	Spring Clean Salad (see page 47)
Dinner	Wheat-free pasta with Red-hot Sauce (see page 58)

THURSDAY

Breakfast	Homemade Muesli (see page 36)
Lunch	Chickpea & Tomato Salad (see page 43) with goat's cheese
Dinner	Stuffed aubergine (see page 48); green salad with Basic Salad Dressing (see page 58)

FRIDAY

Breakfast	Soya Yogurt (see page 37) with mixed berries and 1 tsp sunflower seeds
Lunch	Hummus (see page 38) with oatcakes and raw vegetables
Dinner	Vegetable Chilli (see page 50) with brown rice; Sweetcorn & Tomato Salsa (see page 59)

SATURDAY

Breakfast	Apple, Carrot & Cucumber Juice (see page 37)
Lunch	Grilled Vegetable Soup (see page 40) with wheat-free bread
Dinner	Millet Pilaf (see page 53)

SUNDAY

Breakfast	Tropical Smoothie (see page 37); slice of wheat-free toast with honey
Lunch	Green Pea Dip (see page 38) with raw vegetables and oatcakes; Fresh Fruit Salad (see page 56)
Dinner	Mixed salad with drained canned tuna (Hummus [see page 38] if vegetarian)

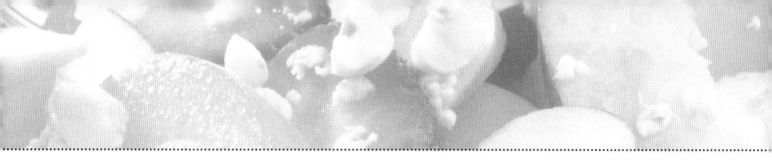

WEEK TWO

MONDAY

Breakfast	Homemade Muesli (see page 36)
Lunch	Spicy Carrot Soup (see page 42) with wheat-free bread
Dinner	Chickpea & Tomato Salad (see page 43) with goat's cheese or smoked tofu; Spicy Baked Apples (see page 56)

TUESDAY

Breakfast	Soya Yogurt (see page 37) with honey and oatmeal
Lunch	Beansprout, Apricot & Almond Salad (see page 45)
Dinner	Tofu & Vegetable Stir-fry (see page 51)

WEDNESDAY

Breakfast	Fresh Fruit Salad (see page 56) with 1 tsp sunflower seeds
Lunch	Ratatouille (see page 55) with wheat-free pasta
Dinner	Squash & Cannellini Bean Soup (see page 41) with wheat-free bread

THURSDAY

Breakfast	Boiled or poached egg with wheat-free toast
Lunch	Spiced Aubergine Soup (see page 42)
Dinner	Asparagus & Tomato Salad (see page 46) with grilled mackerel, trout or sardines (grilled goat's cheese if vegetarian)

FRIDAY

Breakfast	Tropical Smoothie (see page 37)
Lunch	Spring Clean Salad (see page 47)
Dinner	Baked potato with drained canned tuna in oil (Hummus [see page 38] if vegetarian); Red Pepper & Radicchio Salad (see page 47)

SATURDAY

Breakfast	Fresh Fruit Muesli (see page 36)
Lunch	Tomato & Courgette Soup (see page 41)
Dinner	Wheat-free pasta with Red-hot Sauce (see page 58)

SUNDAY

Breakfast	Beetroot, Pear & Spinach Juice (see page 37); wheat-free toast and honey
Lunch	Hummus (see page 38), raw vegetables and oatcakes or ricecakes
Dinner	Vegetable Curry (see page 54)

WEEK THREE

MONDAY

Breakfast Apple, Carrot & Cucumber Juice (see page 37); wheat-free toast and honey

Lunch Hummus (see page 38) and raw vegetables; Beansprout, Apricot & Almond Salad (see page 45)

Dinner Roasted Root Vegetable Stew (see page 53) with brown rice or quinoa; Fruity Nut Bars (see page 57)

TUESDAY

Breakfast Soya Yogurt (see page 37) with mixed fruit and 1 tsp sunflower seeds

Lunch Grilled Vegetable Soup (see page 40) with wheat-free bread; fresh fruit

Dinner Spaghetti with Pecan Nuts & Herbs (see page 54); green salad with Basic Salad Dressing (see page 58)

WEDNESDAY

Breakfast ½ melon filled with berries and 1 tsp sunflower seeds

Lunch Fennel & Orange Salad (see page 44)

Dinner Millet Pilaf (see page 53)

THURSDAY

Breakfast Tropical Smoothie (see page 37)

Lunch Chickpea & Tomato Salad (see page 43) with grilled tofu

Dinner Stuffed courgettes (see page 48); rocket and watercress salad with Basic Salad Dressing (see page 58)

FRIDAY

Breakfast ½ grapefruit; wheat-free toast with honey

Lunch Hummus (see page 38) with raw vegetables; Wild Rice Salad with Cucumber & Orange (see page 47)

Dinner Squash & Cannellini Bean Soup (see page 41) with wheat-free bread; Spring Clean Salad (see page 47)

SATURDAY

Breakfast Fresh Fruit Muesli (see page 36)

Lunch Asparagus & Tomato Salad (see page 46); fresh fruit

Dinner Garden Paella (see page 52); Spicy Baked Apples (see page 56)

SUNDAY

Breakfast Soya Yogurt (see page 37) with mixed fruit and 1 tsp sunflower seeds

Lunch Penne with Broccoli, Peppers & Pine Nuts (see page 50)

Dinner Baked potato with Hummus (see page 38); Sweetcorn & Tomato Salsa (see page 59); mixed leaves and Basic Salad Dressing (see page 58)

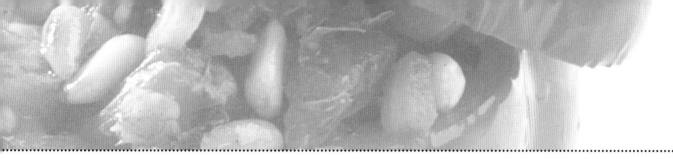

WEEK FOUR

MONDAY

Breakfast Beetroot, Pear & Spinach Juice
(see page 37); wheat-free toast with honey

Lunch Hummus (see page 38) and raw
vegetables; Tomato & Courgette Soup
(see page 41)

Dinner Vegetable Curry (see page 54) with
brown rice

TUESDAY

Breakfast ½ grapefruit; wheat-free toast with honey

Lunch Green Pea Dip (see page 38) with raw
vegetables; Spicy Carrot Soup (see page 42)
with wheat-free bread

Dinner Tofu & Vegetable Stir-fry (see page 51) with
rice noodles

WEDNESDAY

Breakfast Fresh Fruit Muesli (see page 36)

Lunch Squash & Cannellini Bean Soup
(see page 41) with wheat-free bread

Dinner Stuffed Peppers (see page 48); Asparagus &
Tomato Salad (see page 46)

THURSDAY

Breakfast Tropical Smoothie (see page 37)

Lunch Olive, Sun-dried Tomato & Lentil Pâté (see
page 39) with oatcakes or wheat-free bread;
Spring Clean Salad (see page 47)

Dinner Garden Paella (see page 52); green salad
with Basic Salad Dressing (see page 58)

FRIDAY

Breakfast Soya Yogurt (see page 37) with 1 tsp
sunflower seeds and honey

Lunch Spiced Aubergine Soup (see page 42) with
wheat-free bread

Dinner Baked potato and Hummus (see page 38);
Red Pepper & Radicchio Salad (see page 47);
Strawberry Mousse (see page 57)

SATURDAY

Breakfast Homemade Muesli (see page 36)

Lunch Fennel & Orange Salad (see page 44);
Hummus (see page 38) with oatcakes

Dinner Vegetable Chilli (see page 50) with
Sweetcorn & Tomato Salsa (see page 59)
and corn tortillas

SUNDAY

Breakfast Fresh citrus fruits with honey and Soya
Yogurt (see page 37)

Lunch Ratatouille (see page 55) with wheat-free
pasta

Dinner Warm New Potato & Lentil Salad (see page
45); green salad with Basic Salad Dressing
(see page 58); Fruity Nut Bars (see page 57)

BREAKFASTS, JUICES & SMOOTHIES

FRESH FRUIT MUESLI

A winning combination of antioxidant vitamins, protein and essential fatty acids. **Serves 1**

115 g (4 oz) fresh fruit (e.g. apples, strawberries, peaches, apricots)

1 tbsp porridge oats, pre-soaked

1 tbsp water

handful chopped hazelnuts

1 Wash the fresh fruit and trim as necessary. Chop or slice.

2 Mix in the cereal base and water.

3 Sprinkle with chopped hazelnuts.

MUESLI

Figs contain the enzyme ficin, which improves the absorption of other nutrients. **Makes 10 servings**

225 g (8 oz) rolled oats (porridge oats)

85 g (3 oz) each of raw almonds, brazil nuts and hazelnuts

85 g (3 oz) raisins

85 g (3 oz) each of dried figs, apricots and peaches, chopped

25 g (1 oz) sunflower seeds

1 Mix all the ingredients together in a bowl.

2 Serve with apple juice or rice, soya or almond milk.

SEEDS FOR HEALTH

Put one measure each of sesame, sunflower and pumpkin seeds and two measures of flax seeds in a jar. Seal and keep in the fridge. Grind two tablespoons of these seeds in a coffee grinder and add to cereal or yogurt to guarantee a good intake of essential fatty acids.

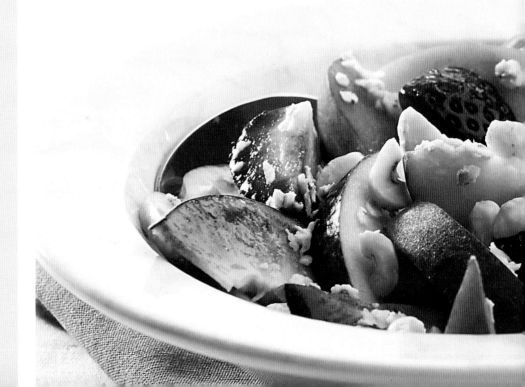

SOYA YOGURT

Live yogurt helps to repopulate the digestive system with friendly bacteria to ensure it runs smoothly. This yogurt is delicious with fresh fruit, fruit purées or honey. Serves 4

600 ml (1 pint) soya milk

4 tbsp powdered soya milk

1 tbsp live natural soya yogurt

1 Boil the soya milk in a saucepan. Leave to cool until tepid. Add the powdered soya milk and yogurt and blend with a hand whisk.

2 Rinse a vacuum flask with boiling water to sterilize it. Pour in the soya mixture, replace the lid and keep in a warm place overnight (an airing cupboard is ideal).

3 Empty the flask contents into smaller pots or jars and refrigerate. Save 1 tablespoon of yogurt to use as a starter next time you make yogurt.

TROPICAL SMOOTHIE

Pineapple and papaya are rich in antioxidants and contain digestive-system stimulating enzymes. Serves 2

1 ripe papaya, peeled, stoned and chopped

½ fresh pineapple, peeled and chopped

150 ml (¼ pint) soya milk

300 ml (½ pint) Soya Yogurt (see left)

Place all the ingredients in a juicer or blender and process until smooth.

APPLE, CARROT & CUCUMBER JUICE

This drink is packed with antioxidants and soluble fibre, and the diuretic properties of cucumber and carrot help relieve fluid retention. Serves 1

1 apple, unpeeled, cored and chopped

1 carrot, peeled and chopped

½ cucumber, chopped

Place the ingredients in a juicer or blender and process.

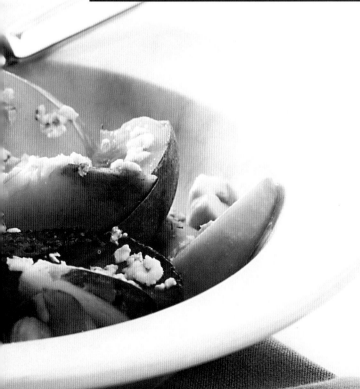

Fresh fruit muesli

BEETROOT, PEAR & SPINACH JUICE

Beetroot stimulates the liver and helps to cleanse the digestive system. The pear adds sweetness and fibre. Spinach contains antioxidants that help to eliminate free radicals. Serves 1

1 beetroot, trimmed, peeled and chopped

1 pear, cored and chopped

25 g (1 oz) fresh spinach leaves

Place the ingredients in a juicer or blender and process. Dilute with filtered water to taste.

DIPS & SPREADS

Serve these versatile dips with an array of colourful raw vegetables, or spread on wheat-free bread.

HUMMUS

Chickpeas are highly nutritious and very versatile.

400 g (14 oz) canned chickpeas, drained and rinsed

2 garlic cloves

2–3 tbsp water

2 tbsp tahini

1 tbsp olive oil

juice of 1 lemon

black pepper

paprika, to garnish

1 Place the chickpeas, garlic, water, tahini, olive oil and lemon juice in a food processor. Process until smooth, adding more water or lemon juice if necessary. Season with black pepper.

2 Transfer into a bowl, cover and refrigerate.

3 To serve, garnish with a sprinkling of paprika.

GREEN PEA DIP

Frozen peas are an excellent source of vitamin C. This dip makes a good substitute for guacamole (avocado spread, which is high in fat).

juice and zest of 1 lime

½ fresh green chilli pepper, deseeded and finely chopped

2 tbsp chopped fresh parsley

1 tbsp chopped fresh coriander

225 g (8 oz) thawed frozen peas

4 spring onions, chopped

1 Place all the ingredients except the lime zest in a food processor and process to a rough purée. If necessary, add a little water to thin the mixture.

2 Spoon into a bowl, cover and refrigerate.

3 To serve, garnish with lime zest.

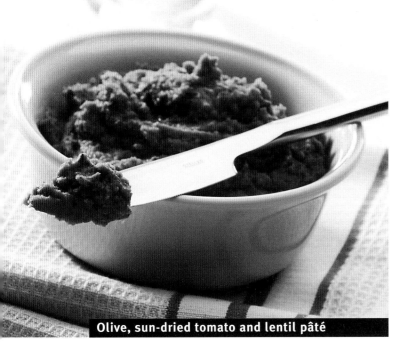

Olive, sun-dried tomato and lentil pâté

OLIVE, SUN-DRIED TOMATO & LENTIL PÂTÉ

This tasty spread is a good source of healthy fats, vitamin C and soluble fibre.

1 garlic clove, crushed

3 spring onions, sliced

½ fresh red chilli, deseeded and finely chopped

2 dry-packed sun-dried tomatoes, chopped

4 black olives, stones removed

225 ml (8 fl oz) vegetable stock

115 g (4 oz) red lentils, rinsed

black pepper

1 Put the garlic, spring onions, chilli, tomatoes and olives in a saucepan with half the stock. Bring to the boil, reduce the heat and simmer until the onions are tender.

2 Stir in the red lentils and the rest of the stock. Simmer for 20 minutes or until the lentils are tender, adding water if necessary to prevent the lentils sticking to the pan. Season with black pepper and leave to cool.

3 Transfer the mixture to a blender and purée until smooth. Spoon into a bowl, cover and refrigerate.

CRUDITÉS

Most vegetables can be eaten raw, and they improve the overall fibre content of a meal when served with one of the dips. Choose a few of the following:

- carrot sticks
- celery sticks
- cucumber sticks
- courgette sticks
- strips of red, green or yellow pepper
- baby sweetcorn
- broccoli or cauliflower florets
- spring onions
- mangetout
- radishes
- tomatoes

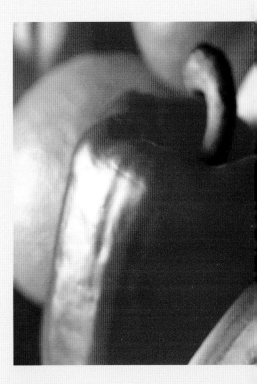

SOUPS

GRILLED VEGETABLE SOUP

This combination of smoky aubergines, red peppers, tomatoes, garlic and herbs makes the quintessential Mediterranean soup, which is packed with vitamins, cleansers and phytonutrients. Serves 4–6

1 onion, halved but not peeled

4 garlic cloves

4 ripe tomatoes

2 aubergines, halved lengthways

2 red peppers, halved and deseeded

1 tbsp olive oil

5 sprigs thyme

1 bay leaf

1 litre (1³/₄ pints) vegetable stock

sun-dried tomatoes, chopped

¹/₂ lemon, freshly squeezed

black pepper

handful basil leaves, torn, to serve

1 Place the onion, garlic, tomatoes, aubergines and peppers under a preheated hot grill for 10 minutes until charred and softened. Leave to cool slightly, then peel the onion, garlic and tomatoes. Remove any charred skin from the aubergines and peppers. Roughly chop.

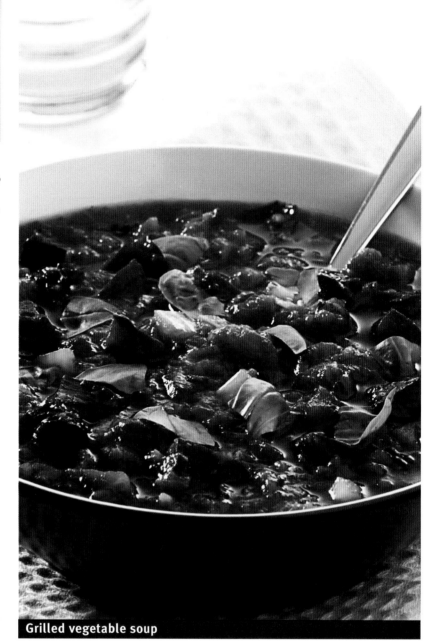

Grilled vegetable soup

2 Gently heat the olive oil with the thyme and bay leaf in a large, heavy-based saucepan for 2 minutes. Add the chopped vegetables, sun-dried tomatoes and stock. Bring to the boil, cover and simmer gently for 20 minutes.

3 Leave to cool then remove the bay leaf. Transfer the soup to a food processor and process briefly to retain some of the vegetables' texture.

4 Return the soup to the pan, season with lemon juice and pepper and reheat.

5 To serve, garnish with torn basil leaves.

SQUASH & CANNELLINI BEAN SOUP

This nutritious soup is packed with the antioxidant vitamins A, C and E. Serves 4

1 red pepper, halved and deseeded

1 litre (1³/₄ pints) vegetable stock

1 onion, finely chopped

2 garlic cloves, crushed

1 butternut squash, peeled and diced

450 g (1 lb) sweet potatoes, peeled and diced

1 tsp chopped sage

1 bay leaf

400 g (14 oz) canned cannellini beans, drained and rinsed

1 tsp olive oil

juice of ¹/₂ lemon

black pepper

1 Place the pepper skin-side upwards under a very hot grill until blackened. Place in a plastic bag and leave to cool slightly, then remove the skin and cut the pepper into very thin strips.

2 Heat a little of the stock in a large saucepan and gently sauté the onion and garlic for a few minutes until softened. Add the squash and sweet potatoes and cook for 5 minutes.

3 Add the red pepper, rest of the stock and herbs and bring to the boil. Reduce the heat, cover and simmer for 30 minutes or until the vegetables are tender.

4 Remove the bay leaf. Add the beans, olive oil and lemon juice and season with black pepper. Cook for a further 5 minutes then serve hot.

TOMATO & COURGETTE SOUP

Tomatoes form the base of many vegetable soups. As well as being a good source of vitamin C they contain the powerful antioxidant lycopene. Courgettes are diuretic; garlic and onion are rich in sulphur, which binds with toxins to remove them from the body. Basil stimulates the circulation.
Serves 4

450 g (1 lb) ripe tomatoes

1 litre (1³/₄ pints) vegetable stock

1 onion, finely chopped

2 garlic cloves, finely chopped

black pepper

225 g (8 oz) courgettes

1 tsp olive oil

handful fresh basil leaves, roughly chopped, to serve

1 Using a sharp knife, make crosses in the tops of the tomatoes and put them into a heatproof bowl. Pour over boiling water and leave for 2 minutes. Drain the tomatoes, then skin them, chop finely and leave to one side.

2 Heat a little of the vegetable stock in a heavy saucepan and gently sauté the onion and garlic until translucent. Add the chopped tomatoes and rest of the stock. Bring to the boil, cover and simmer gently for 20 minutes. Season to taste with pepper. Cut the courgettes into small cubes, add to the soup and bring to boiling point. Allow to bubble for 2 minutes until the courgettes are just tender. Drizzle in the olive oil.

3 To serve, ladle into a bowl and sprinkle the basil leaves on top.

SPICED AUBERGINE SOUP

This soup, based on flavours used widely in Middle Eastern cooking, is very good for eliminating excess fluid. **Serves 4**

1 aubergine, halved

2 tbsp vegetable stock

1 red onion, chopped

2 cloves garlic, roughly chopped

half bird's-eye chilli, deseeded and finely chopped

1 tsp ground cumin

1 tsp paprika

handful fresh coriander

handful fresh mint leaves, plus extra to garnish

1 tsp olive oil

1/2 lemon, freshly squeezed

black pepper

125 ml (4 fl oz) Soya Yogurt (see page 37), plus extra for garnish

1 cucumber, peeled and diced

1   Grill the aubergine under a high heat for 10 minutes, turning until the skins are blackened. Leave to cool.

2   Heat the vegetable stock in a frying pan over a low heat. Add the onion, garlic, chilli and ground spices. Stir until the onions and garlic are softened, but do not burn.

3   Scrape the flesh off the aubergine into a strainer and use the back of a spoon to press out as much liquid as possible. Put the aubergine, onion, garlic, chilli, ground spices, coriander, mint, olive oil and lemon juice into a food processor and whizz into a smooth purée.

4   Turn into a mixing bowl and season to taste with black pepper. Stir in the yogurt and the diced cucumber, then put the bowl in the refrigerator to chill.

5   Serve with a swirl of soya yogurt and a sprig of mint.

SPICY CARROT SOUP

Old carrots in particular are an excellent source of beta-carotene, which your body converts to the antioxidant vitamin A. Ginger stimulates blood flow to the tiniest vessels in your body. **Serves 4**

1 onion, chopped

1 garlic clove, chopped

1 litre (1³/₄ pints) vegetable stock

675 g (1¹/₂ lb) carrots, chopped

1 tsp freshly grated ginger root

1 tbsp chopped coriander

1   Sauté the onion and garlic in a little of the stock until the onions are translucent. Add the carrots and ginger. Cover the pan and cook for 5 minutes, stirring occasionally.

2   Add the rest of the stock, bring to the boil then reduce the heat and simmer for about 15 minutes or until the carrots are tender.

3   Pour the mixture into a blender and purée. Return to the pan and reheat. Serve, garnished with coriander.

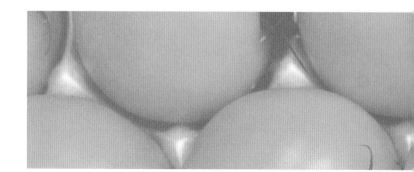

SALADS

CHICKPEA & TOMATO SALAD

Chickpeas are high in protein, phosphorus, sulphur and potassium. Serve with cubes of grilled smoked tofu or goat's cheese for a complete meal. Serves 4

175 g (6 oz) chickpeas or 400 g (14 oz) canned, drained and rinsed

1 green chilli, deseeded and finely chopped

1 garlic clove, crushed

juice and zest of 2 lemons

2 tbsp olive oil

1 tbsp water

black pepper

225 g (8 oz) ripe tomatoes, roughly chopped

1 red onion, thinly sliced

handful fresh basil leaves, torn

1 cos or romaine lettuce, torn

1 If using dried chickpeas, soak overnight then boil for at least 30 minutes until soft. Leave to cool.

2 Put the chilli, garlic, lemon juice, olive oil, water and black pepper in a screwtop jar and shake vigorously. Taste and add more lemon juice or oil if necessary.

3 Add the tomatoes, onion and basil to the chickpeas and mix gently. Pour over the dressing and mix again. To serve, arrange on a bed of lettuce.

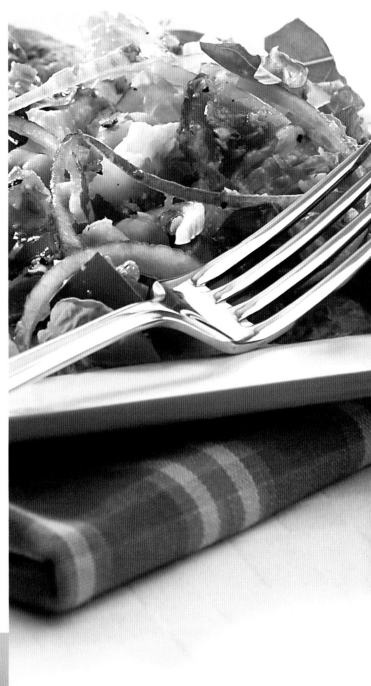

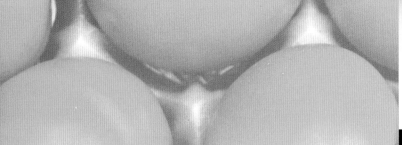

Chickpea & tomato salad

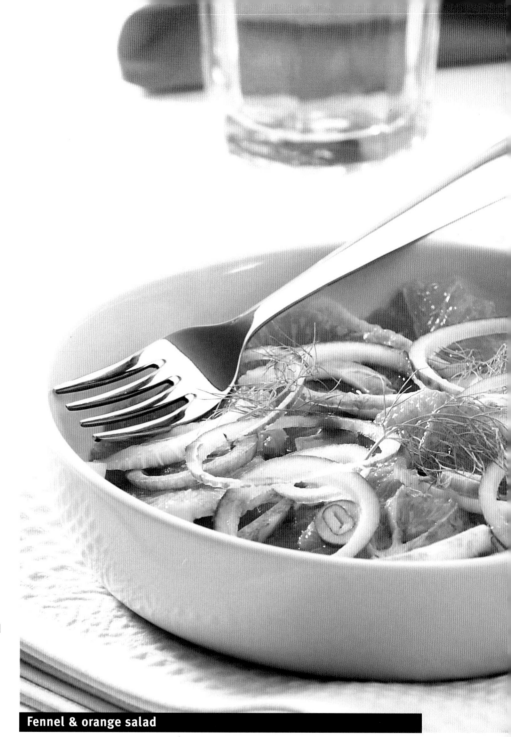

FENNEL & ORANGE SALAD

Fennel stimulates the liver, improves fat digestion and contains essential oils that help get rid of excess fluid.

Serves 4

2 oranges, peeled and sliced

1 bulb Florence fennel, thinly sliced

1 red onion, peeled and sliced into thin rings

juice of 1 orange

2 tbsp balsamic vinegar

1 Arrange the orange slices in the bottom of a shallow dish. Place a layer of fennel on top and then add a layer of onion.

2 Mix the orange juice with the vinegar and drizzle over the salad.

Fennel & orange salad

WARM NEW POTATO & LENTIL SALAD

This nutritious dish can be served as a main course.

Serves 4

85 g (3 oz) puy lentils

450 g (1 lb) new potatoes

6 spring onions

1 tbsp olive oil

2 tbsp balsamic vinegar

black pepper and sea salt

1 Bring a large pan of water to the boil. Rinse the lentils then cook for about 20 minutes or until tender. Drain, rinse and leave to one side.

2 Meanwhile, steam or boil the potatoes until they are soft right through. Drain and halve.

3 Trim the base from the spring onions and cut in long strips.

4 Put the lentils, potatoes and spring onions into a serving dish and toss with the olive oil and vinegar. Season with plenty of black pepper and a little sea salt if required.

BEANSPROUT, APRICOT & ALMOND SALAD

This sweet-tasting salad is packed with antioxidants and helps keep the circulatory system healthy. Beansprouts are rich in vitamin E, apricots are an excellent source of iron, and almonds provide protein and essential fatty acids.

Serves 4

115 g (4 oz) beansprouts, washed and dried

small bunch seedless black and green grapes, halved

12 unsulphured dried apricots, halved

1 tbsp walnut oil

1 tsp sesame oil

2 tsp balsamic vinegar

25 g (1 oz) blanched almonds, halved

black pepper

1 Place the beansprouts in the bottom of a large salad bowl and sprinkle the grapes and apricots on top.

2 Place the oils and vinegar in a screwtop jar and shake vigorously to mix. Pour over the salad.

3 Scatter over the almonds and season with freshly ground black pepper.

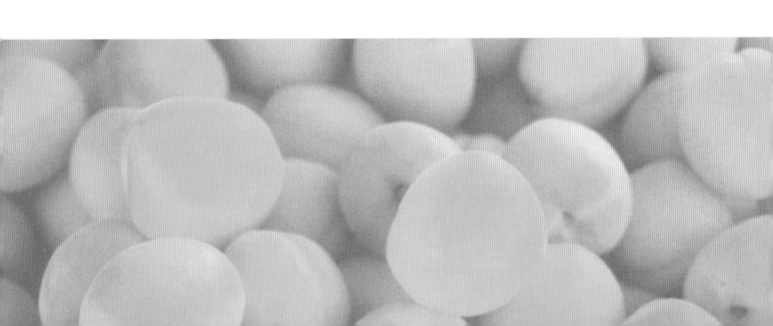

ASPARAGUS & TOMATO SALAD

Asparagus is a gentle diuretic and a kidney stimulant; tomatoes are rich in lycopene, an antioxidant which also protects the heart and blood vessels; watercress protects the lungs and is rich in iron. Serves 4

225 g (8 oz) asparagus spears

1 lamb's lettuce, washed and torn

25 g (1 oz) rocket or mizuna leaves

450 g (1 lb) ripe tomatoes, sliced

12 black olives, stoned and chopped

1 tbsp toasted pine nuts

1 tsp lemon oil

1 tbsp olive oil

1 tsp wholegrain mustard

2 tbsp balsamic vinegar

sea salt and black pepper

1 Steam the asparagus spears for about 8 minutes or until tender. Rinse under cold running water to prevent them cooking any further, then cut into 5-cm (2-in) pieces.

2 Arrange the lettuce and rocket leaves around a salad platter to form the base of the salad. Place the sliced tomatoes in a circle on top and the asparagus in the centre.

3 Sprinkle the black olives and pine nuts over the top. Put the lemon oil, olive oil, mustard and vinegar in a screwtop jar and season to taste with sea salt and black pepper. Shake vigorously and drizzle over the salad.

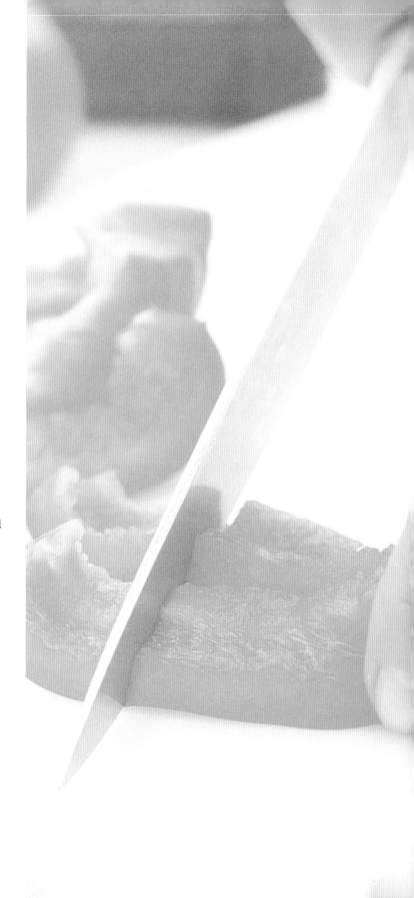

RED PEPPER & RADICCHIO SALAD

This fiery salad boosts the immune system, improves fat digestion and strengthens the blood. Radishes stimulate the digestive organs, beetroot and spring onions benefit the blood and circulation, while the red peppers are excellent antioxidants. Serves 4

> 2 red peppers
>
> 1 head radicchio, separated into leaves
>
> 4 cooked whole beetroot, cut into matchsticks
>
> 12 radishes, sliced
>
> 4 spring onions, finely chopped
>
> 4 tbsp Basic Salad Dressing (see page 58)

1 Core and deseed the peppers and cut into rounds.
2 Arrange the radicchio leaves in a salad bowl. Add the pepper, beetroot, radishes and spring onions. Drizzle with dressing.

SPRING CLEAN SALAD

This diuretic salad is excellent for relieving fluid retention. Serves 4

> 2 dessert apples, cored and diced
>
> juice of 1 lemon
>
> large chunk of watermelon, deseeded and cubed
>
> 1 bulb chicory, sliced into rounds
>
> 4 sticks celery with leaves, roughly chopped
>
> 1 tbsp walnut oil

1 Core and dice the apples, place in a bowl and pour over the lemon juice. Mix well to prevent discolouration.
2 Add the rest of the fruit and vegetables to the bowl and mix gently. Pour in the walnut oil and mix again.

WILD RICE SALAD WITH CUCUMBER & ORANGE

Wild rice is a nutty flavoured type of grass seed. Orange is a powerful cleanser and cucumber relieves water retention. Serves 4

> 225 g (8 oz) wild rice
>
> 850 ml (1½ pints) water
>
> 1 garlic clove, crushed
>
> 1 tbsp balsamic vinegar
>
> 2 tbsp olive oil
>
> sea salt and black pepper
>
> 1 each of red, yellow and orange peppers, skinned, deseeded and thinly sliced
>
> ½ cucumber
>
> 1 orange, peeled, pith removed and cubed
>
> 3 ripe tomatoes cut into chunks
>
> 1 red onion, chopped very finely
>
> generous handful chopped flat-leaf parsley

1 Put the wild rice and water into a large pan and bring to the boil. Stir, cover and simmer for about 40 minutes or until the rice is *al dente* (firm to the bite). Uncover the rice for the last few minutes of cooking to allow any excess water to evaporate.
2 To make the dressing, put the crushed garlic, vinegar, olive oil and seasoning into a screwtop jar and shake vigorously. Add extra vinegar, oil or seasoning as required.
3 Drain the rice and turn into a large bowl. Pour over the dressing and mix in. Then mix in the chopped peppers, cucumber, orange, tomatoes, red onion and flat-leaf parsley.

MAIN DISHES

STUFFED VEGETABLES

This recipe makes a basic nutritious
and cleansing mixture that can be
used to stuff aubergines, courgettes,
tomatoes and peppers. Depending
on the size of the vegetable, this is
enough filling for 2 peppers or
2 medium aubergines.

2 tbsp vegetable stock

1 small onion, chopped

2 garlic cloves, crushed

1 tbsp tomato purée

**6 ripe tomatoes, skinned
(see page 41) and chopped**

4 tbsp cooked brown rice

**25 g (1 oz) pine nuts,
lightly toasted**

1 tbsp chopped fresh parsley

1 tbsp chopped fresh mint

1 tbsp chopped fresh basil

¼ tsp ground cinnamon

juice of 1 lemon

black pepper

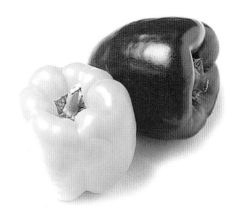

1 Preheat the oven to 180°C/350°F (Gas Mark 4).

•• If stuffing aubergines or courgettes, trim the stems, then halve lengthways.
Use a teaspoon to hollow out each half, leaving a shell about 1 cm (½ in) thick.
Chop the scooped-out flesh. Steam the shells over boiling water for about
4 minutes, then hold under cold water to stop further cooking and dry with
kitchen paper. Mist the insides with oil-and-water spray.

•• If stuffing peppers, slice off the tops (put to one side) and scoop out and
discard the seeds.

•• If stuffing tomatoes, slice off the tops (put to one side), scoop out the seeds
and flesh, and add the latter to the rice mixture in step 2.

2 Heat the stock in a frying pan, add the onions and garlic and sauté, stirring,
until translucent. Stir in the tomato purée, tomatoes, chopped aubergine or
courgette flesh (if using), cooked rice, pine nuts, herbs and cinnamon and
continue cooking for a couple of minutes.

3 Stir in the lemon juice and season with pepper.

4 Lightly mist a baking dish with oil-and-water spray. Stuff the vegetables with
the rice mixture and put the lids back on the peppers or tomatoes. Bake for
about 20 minutes.

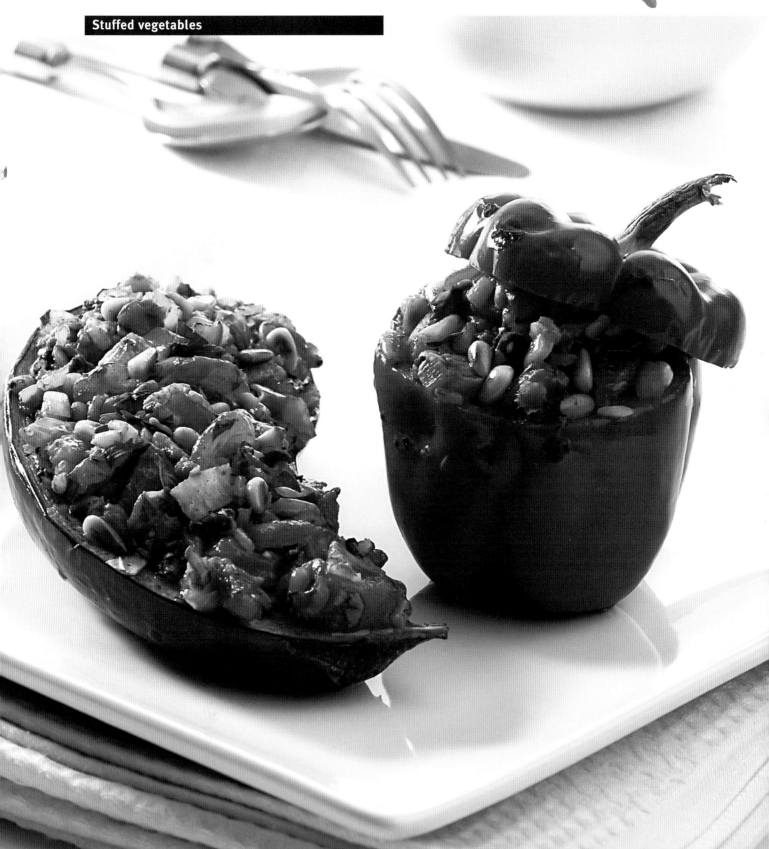

PENNE WITH BROCCOLI, PEPPERS & PINE NUTS

This nutritious recipe contains plenty of antioxidant vitamins and is quick to prepare. Serves 4

1 red and 1 yellow pepper, deseeded and quartered

350 g (12 oz) wheat-free penne pasta

1 head broccoli, divided into florets

1/2 onion, finely chopped

2 garlic cloves, crushed

2 tbsp vegetable stock

1 tbsp tomato purée

25 g (1 oz) pine nuts

12 black olives, stoned and sliced

1 tbsp shredded fresh basil, plus extra to garnish

black pepper

1 Place the peppers under a hot grill and grill, skin-side up, until the skin begins to char. Leave to cool slightly then remove the skin and cut into strips.

2 Fill a large saucepan with water and bring it to the boil. Cook the pasta according to the instructions on the packet, then drain.

3 Steam the broccoli for 5 minutes until just tender.

4 Sauté the onions and garlic in the stock for about 5 minutes or until the onion is translucent. Stir in the red pepper then mix in the tomato purée. Add the broccoli, pine nuts, olives and basil, and season with black pepper. Heat gently for 2 minutes, then stir in the pasta.

5 Transfer to a serving dish and garnish with torn basil leaves.

VEGETABLE CHILLI

This versatile dish can be served with rice or used to stuff corn tortillas and served with salad. Beans are rich sources of protein, B vitamins, minerals, carbohydrates and fibre. Serves 4

1 onion, chopped

2 garlic cloves, crushed

1/2 fresh chilli, deseeded and chopped

300 ml (1/2 pint) vegetable stock

1 tbsp paprika

1 tbsp tomato purée

1 potato, peeled and cubed

2 carrots, chopped

1 courgette, chopped

115 g (4 oz) green beans, sliced

1 red and 1 green pepper, deseeded and chopped

400 g (14 oz) canned chopped tomatoes

400 g (14 oz) canned cannellini beans, drained and rinsed

black pepper

chopped fresh coriander, to garnish

1 Sauté the onion, garlic and chilli in a little of the stock for 5 minutes. Stir in the paprika and tomato purée.

2 Stir in the vegetables and add the chopped tomatoes and the rest of the stock. Bring to the boil, reduce the heat and simmer for about 15 minutes.

3 Add the cannellini beans and simmer for a further 10 minutes.

4 Season with black pepper. Garnish with fresh coriander and serve on a bed of brown rice.

TOFU & VEGETABLE STIR-FRY

Tofu is an excellent source of protein but needs spicing up as it can taste very bland. The liquid added at the end provides a burst of steam to finish off the cooking. Serves 4

2 tbsp vegetable stock

4 spring onions, chopped

2 garlic cloves, crushed

2.5-cm (1-in) piece fresh ginger, peeled and grated

½ fresh red chilli, deseeded and finely chopped

1 red and 1 yellow pepper, deseeded and sliced

115 g (4 oz) green beans, sliced

1 head broccoli, divided into florets

115 g (4 oz) beansprouts, rinsed

225 g (8 oz) firm tofu, cubed

2 tbsp water

juice of 1 lemon

2 tsp sesame oil

55 g (2 oz) blanched almonds, halved

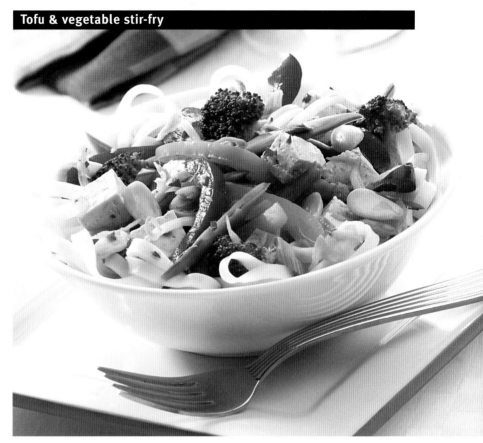

Tofu & vegetable stir-fry

1 Heat the vegetable stock in a wok and stir-fry the onions, garlic, ginger and chilli for 2 minutes.

2 Add the vegetables and stir-fry for 3–4 minutes. Add the tofu and cook for a further 2 minutes.

3 Mix the water and lemon juice together, pour over the vegetables and cook for 1 minute.

4 Stir in the sesame oil and almonds and serve immediately on a bed of rice or rice noodles.

Mediterranean Stir-fries

Stir-fries are associated with Oriental cooking but for an Italian-style stir-fry try a combination of cauliflower, fennel, black olives and red peppers, or courgettes with sultanas, olives, red peppers, lemon juice, fresh parsley and 1 tablespoon of drained, rinsed capers.

GARDEN PAELLA

Short-grain brown rice provides a creamy texture for this Spanish-style dish. Pumpkin seeds are one of the richest sources of zinc, essential for the structure and elasticity of skin.

Serves 4

600 ml (1 pint) vegetable stock

1 onion, finely chopped

2 garlic cloves, crushed

200 g (8 oz) short-grain brown rice

115 g (4 oz) peas, fresh or frozen

115 g (4 oz) green beans, sliced

4 artichoke hearts, halved

6 strands saffron

6 tomatoes, skinned (see page 41) and chopped

1 tsp dried oregano

1 tbsp fresh chopped thyme

2 tbsp finely chopped fresh parsley, plus extra to garnish

black pepper

juice of 1 lemon

12 black or green olives, halved

2 tbsp pumpkin seeds

lemon wedges, to garnish

1 Heat a little of the stock in a large saucepan and sauté the onion and garlic until soft.

2 Add the rice and cook gently for 1 minute. Add the peas, beans and artichoke hearts, stirring well, and cook over a very low heat for 4–5 minutes.

3 Bring the rest of the stock to boil in another pan, dissolve the saffron in the boiling stock, then add to the paella pan with the tomatoes and herbs.

4 Bring to the boil, reduce the heat and cook, uncovered, for about 30 minutes, stirring frequently. Add more liquid if necessary.

5 Season with black pepper and add the lemon juice. Stir in the olives and pumpkin seeds, garnish with chopped parsley and lemon wedges, and serve hot.

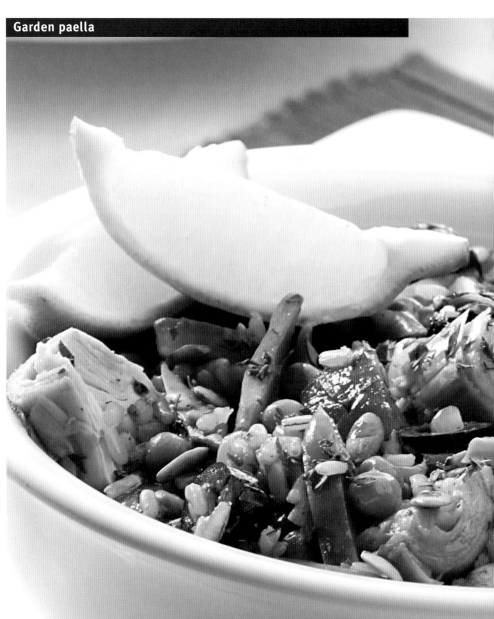

Garden paella

MILLET PILAF

Broad beans are a good source of protein, selenium, zinc, potassium and iron. Serves 4

300 ml (½ pint) vegetable stock

1 onion, chopped

1 garlic clove, crushed

6 cardamom pods

1 stick cinnamon

2 bay leaves

175 g (6 oz) millet

115 g (4 oz) frozen broad beans

115 g (4 oz) peas, fresh or frozen

black pepper

55 g (2 oz) sunflower seeds

2 tbsp finely chopped fresh parsley

1 tbsp finely chopped fresh mint

1 Sauté the onion and garlic in a little of the vegetable stock for about 5 minutes until soft. Add the spices and bay leaves and cook over a moderate heat for 2 minutes.

2 Remove the spices and bay leaves with a slotted spoon and discard. Add the millet and pour over the rest of the stock. Bring to the boil, cover and reduce the heat until it is cooking gently.

3 Leave to simmer for about 20 minutes, checking to make sure it does not stick to the pan and adding more water if necessary.

4 Add the broad beans and peas and cook for a further 5 minutes.

5 Season with black pepper and stir in the sunflower seeds, parsley, and mint.

ROASTED ROOT VEGETABLE STEW

Root vegetables are a powerhouse of immune-enhancing nutrients. Fennel helps maintain hormone balance and rids the body of excess fluid. Serves 4

3 garlic cloves, peeled

1 onion, cut into wedges

1 parsnip, peeled and sliced

2 carrots, peeled and sliced

1 butternut squash or small pumpkin, peeled and sliced

1 fennel bulb, halved and sliced

1 sweet potato, peeled and cubed

1 tbsp olive oil

300 ml (½ pint) vegetable stock

1 tbsp chopped fresh tarragon

1 tbsp wholegrain mustard

1 tbsp tomato purée

juice of 1 lemon

black pepper

1 Preheat the oven to 200°C/400°F (Gas Mark 6).

2 Spread all the vegetables in a large roasting tin and pour over the oil and half the stock. Stir to combine.

3 Bake, uncovered, for about 30 minutes until the vegetables are tender, stirring occasionally.

4 Reduce the oven temperature to 180°C/350°F (Gas Mark 4). In a bowl or measuring jug, mix the remaining stock with the tarragon, mustard, tomato purée, lemon juice and black pepper. Stir into the vegetables and bake for a further 15 minutes. Serve with brown rice and a bean salad.

VEGETABLE CURRY

Lentils are rich in protein, an excellent source of iron and also contain B vitamins. The vitamin C in the vegetables improves the absorption of iron; and the diuretic properties of the fennel, celery and parsley will make sure your body eliminates waste products effectively. Serves 4

> 1 onion, finely chopped
>
> 2 garlic cloves, crushed
>
> 1 tsp ground cumin
>
> 1 tsp ground ginger
>
> 1 tsp ground turmeric
>
> 1 tsp ground chilli
>
> 600 ml (1 pint) vegetable stock
>
> 2 sticks celery, sliced
>
> 2 carrots, peeled and chopped
>
> 1 red and 1 green pepper, deseeded and chopped
>
> 1 bulb fennel, cut into 1-cm (1/2-in) slices
>
> 2 courgettes, sliced
>
> 1 head broccoli, divided into florets
>
> 115 g (4 oz) red or green lentils
>
> juice of 1 lemon
>
> black pepper
>
> 4 tbsp chopped fresh parsley
>
> 2 tbsp chopped fresh coriander

1 Put the onion, garlic, spices and half the stock in a heavy-bottomed saucepan. Cover, bring to the boil and cook for 5 minutes, until the onions and garlic are translucent. Stir in the celery, carrots, peppers and fennel, reduce the heat and simmer, stirring frequently, for 5 minutes.

2 Stir in the courgettes, broccoli, lentils and lemon juice and add the rest of the stock. Season with black pepper, cover and simmer gently for about 20 minutes or until the vegetables and lentils are tender.

3 Stir in the fresh herbs just before serving, add a pinch of sea salt if necessary and serve with brown rice.

SPAGHETTI WITH PECAN NUTS & HERBS

This simple dish can be made with chopped walnuts instead of pecans. Parsley is a diuretic and garlic and basil are excellent for the circulation. Serves 4

> 55 g (2 oz) shelled pecan nuts
>
> 2 tbsp vegetable stock
>
> 2 garlic cloves, crushed
>
> 1 red chilli, deseeded and finely sliced
>
> handful of flat-leaf parsley, finely chopped
>
> black pepper
>
> 12 leaves fresh basil, shredded
>
> 225 g (8 oz) wheat-free spaghetti

1 Put the pecan nuts in a food processor or blender and grind roughly.

2 Heat the vegetable stock in a pan and sauté the garlic, chilli and parsley for 1 minute. Add the nuts and continue stirring for about a minute, being careful not to let them brown. Season with black pepper and remove from the heat. Mix in the basil leaves.

3 Bring a pan of water to the boil, cook the spaghetti according to the instructions on the packet and drain.

4 Mix the pecan mixture in thoroughly and transfer to a serving bowl.

RATATOUILLE

This classic medley of Mediterranean flavours is packed with vitamins and antibacterial essential oils, and is delicious tossed with wheat-free pasta or on a bed of buckwheat. Serves 4

2 red peppers, deseeded and quartered

2 tbsp vegetable stock

1 onion, very thinly sliced

3 garlic cloves, crushed

2 aubergines, diced

3 courgettes, sliced

400 g (14 oz) canned chopped tomatoes

leaves from a few sprigs each of thyme, marjoram and oregano

black pepper

2 tsp olive oil

handful of chopped flat-leaf parsley

handful of shredded basil leaves

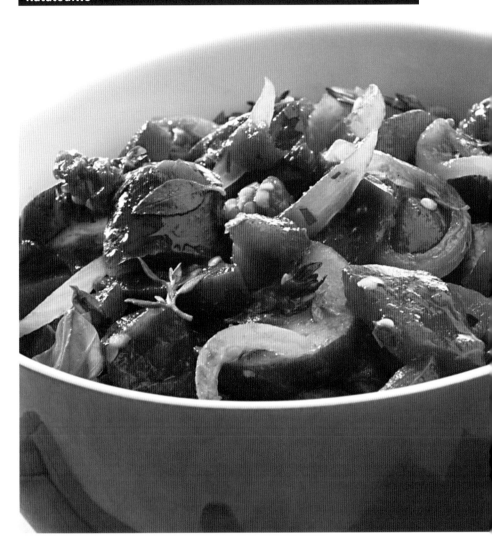

Ratatouille

1   Place the peppers under a hot grill and grill, skin-side up, until the skin begins to char. Leave to cool slightly then remove the skin and cut into chunks.

2   Heat the vegetable stock and sauté the onion and garlic until translucent. Add the aubergines and courgettes, and continue to cook for about 5 minutes. Mix in the red peppers and cook, stirring occasionally, for another minute.

3   Add the tomatoes and snip in the thyme, marjoram and oregano leaves. Season with black pepper.

4   Cover and simmer for about 40 minutes. Stir in the olive oil, parsley and basil and cook, uncovered, for a further 10 minutes until there is no surplus liquid.

DESSERTS

FRESH FRUIT SALAD

This colourful fruit salad is simply bursting with vitamins and antioxidants. Serves 4

**1 ripe mango or papaya,
or 2 peaches or nectarines**

1 pineapple

2 kiwi fruit

115 g (4 oz) strawberries, hulled

115 g (4 oz) each of green and black seedless grapes

juice of 1 lemon

4 tbsp apple juice

1 Prepare the fruit by peeling the mango, pineapple and kiwi fruit over a large bowl to collect the juices. Sliver the fruit into the bowl.

2 Halve the strawberries and grapes into the bowl.

3 Pour over the lemon juice and apple juice and mix gently. Refrigerate for several hours to allow the juices to combine before serving.

SPICY BAKED APPLES

One of the main benefits of apples is their high content of the soluble fibre pectin, which helps lower cholesterol and improves digestion. For variety, use pears instead. Serves 4

4 Bramley apples, cored

55 g (2 oz) dried mixed fruit

1 tsp honey

½ tsp ground ginger

½ tsp ground cinnamon

1 Preheat the oven to 190°C/375°F (Gas Mark 5).

2 Place the apples in an ovenproof dish.

3 Mix the dried fruit, honey and spices and stuff the apple cavities with the mixture. Put 4 tbsp water in the dish, cover with foil and bake for about 30 minutes or until tender.

4 Serve hot with Soya Yogurt (see page 37) spooned over.

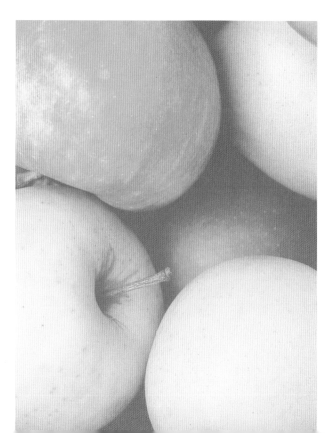

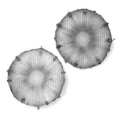

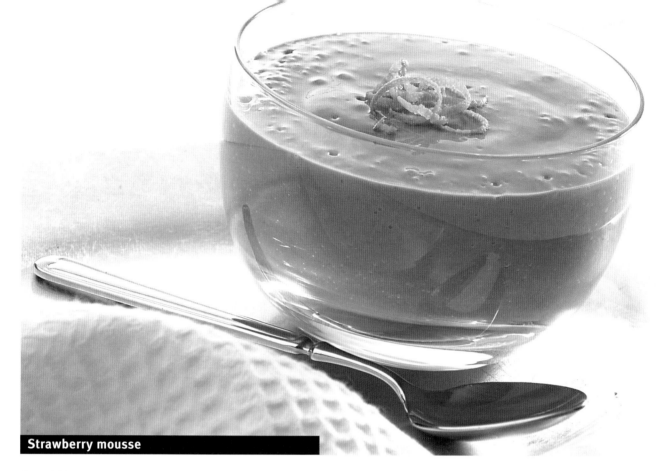

Strawberry mousse

STRAWBERRY MOUSSE

Not only are strawberries full of vitamin C, but the natural substances that give them their colour are powerful antioxidants. Other berries such as black cherries, blueberries and blackcurrants can be used instead. Serves 4

225 g (8 oz) silken tofu

450 g (1 lb) ripe strawberries, hulled, washed and dried

zest of 1 orange

1 tsp honey

1   Drain the tofu and place in a food processor or blender.

2   Roughly chop the strawberries and put in the food processor. Reserve some of the orange zest strips for decoration, and put the remaining zest in the food processor with the honey.

3   Process until smooth, spoon into dessert dishes and chill in the refrigerator.

4   Decorate with the reserved orange zest.

FRUITY NUT BARS

Dates and apricots are excellent sources of iron and the nuts provide essential fatty acids and proteins. Serves 4

55 g (2 oz) unsulphured dried apricots

55 g (2 oz) dates, stoned

55 g (2 oz) raisins

55 g (2 oz) sunflower seeds

55 g (2 oz) hazelnuts

115 g (4 oz) porridge oats

juice of 1 lemon

1 tbsp apple juice

1   Preheat the oven to 180°C/350°F (Gas Mark 4).

2   Finely chop the dried fruit and nuts and mix with the other ingredients.

3   Line an 18-cm (7-inch) baking tin with greaseproof paper. Press the mixture into the tin and bake for about 15 minutes.

4   Cut into slices while still warm.

DRESSING, SALSA & SAUCE

BASIC SALAD DRESSING

This dressing will keep for a few days in a dark, tightly stoppered bottle and is perfect for any salad. The olive oil, garlic, rosemary and cider vinegar are extremely beneficial for the circulatory and digestive systems.

> **200 ml (7 fl oz) olive oil**
>
> **115 ml (4 fl oz) cider vinegar**
>
> **2 tbsp water**
>
> **1 tbsp honey**
>
> **1 tbsp wholegrain mustard**
>
> **1 garlic clove, finely chopped**
>
> **1 sprig rosemary**
>
> **pinch of sea salt and freshly ground black pepper**

Place all the ingredients in a screwtop jar and shake well. Taste, adding more mustard, vinegar or seasoning as you prefer. This recipe makes about 300 ml (½ pint) dressing but you can make any quantity you like, as long as the proportions are the same.

RED-HOT SAUCE

This is rich in detoxifying ingredients and perfect for dressing up wheat-free pasta. Serves 4

> **2 tbsp vegetable stock**
>
> **1 small onion, finely chopped**
>
> **2 garlic cloves, crushed**
>
> **1–2 fresh red chillies, according to taste, deseeded and finely chopped**
>
> **1 tbsp tomato purée**
>
> **400 g (14 oz) canned chopped tomatoes**
>
> **handful parsley, stalks removed, finely chopped**
>
> **handful basil, shredded, plus a couple of extra sprigs to garnish**
>
> **12 olives, stoned and sliced**
>
> **juice of 1 lemon**
>
> **black pepper**

1. Heat the vegetable stock in a medium-sized pan and sauté the onion, garlic and chilli for a few minutes. Stir in the tomato purée and add the chopped tomatoes. Simmer for 5 minutes. Stir in the herbs and cook for a further 5 minutes.

2. Stir in the olives and cook for 2 minutes. Add the lemon juice and black pepper to taste. Garnish with basil and serve with cooked wheat-free pasta.

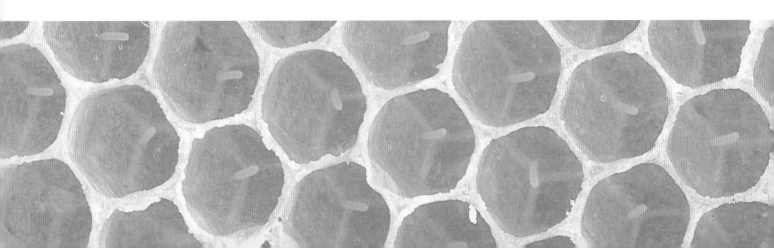

SWEETCORN & TOMATO SALSA

This salsa contains many substances that cleanse the body and stimulate the circulation. Serves 4

115 g (4 oz) frozen sweetcorn

¹/₂ red onion, finely chopped

¹/₂ red chilli, deseeded and finely chopped

115 g (4 oz) ripe tomatoes, chopped

¹/₂ cucumber, chopped

4 radishes, sliced

1 tbsp fresh basil, roughly shredded

juice of 1 lime

black pepper

1 Cook the sweetcorn according to the packet instructions and leave to cool.

2 Mix all the ingredients together, cover and leave to stand at room temperature for at least an hour before serving.

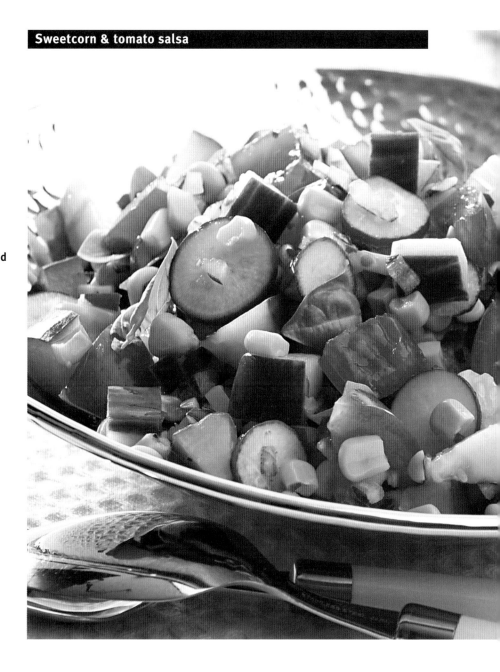

Sweetcorn & tomato salsa

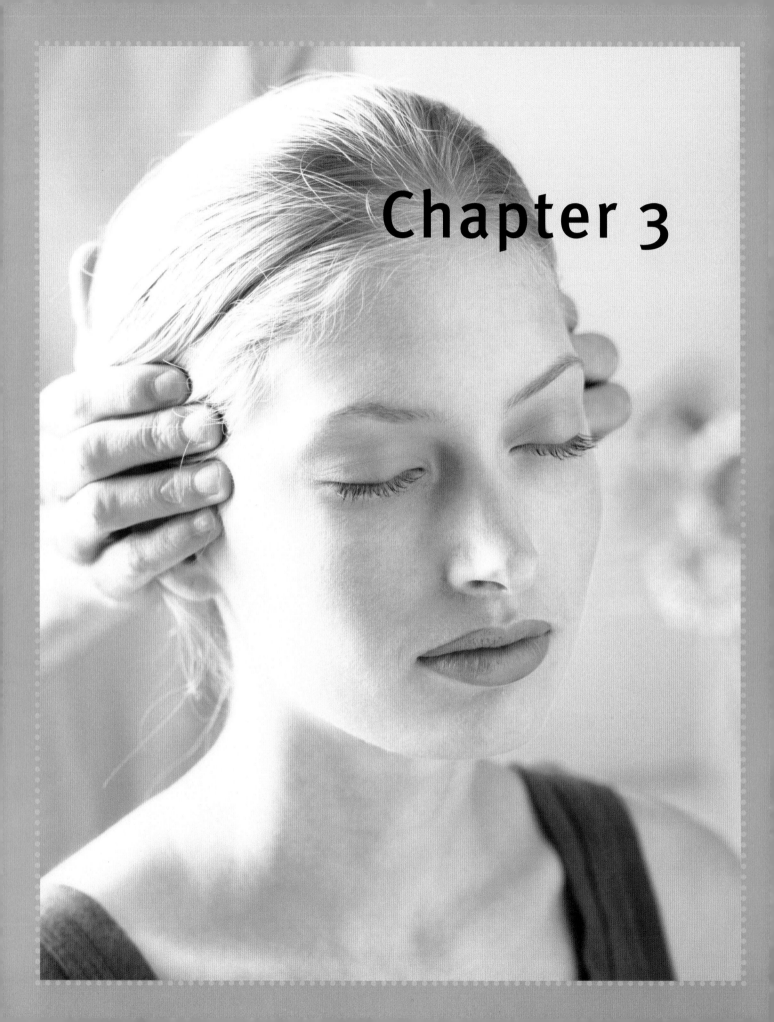

Chapter 3

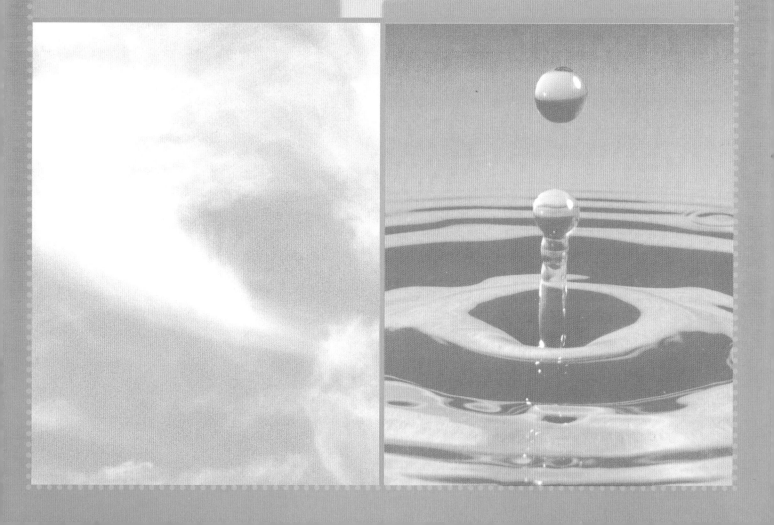

BODY & MIND DETOX

Daily schedule

- 5 minutes: skin brushing
- 5 minutes: shower or bath
- 20 minutes: exercise
- 10–20 minutes: relaxation
  therapies, such as meditation,
  visualization, progressive muscle
  relaxation and deep breathing

Weekly schedule

- Exfoliation
- Facial
- Scalp massage and hair mask
- Hand and foot massage

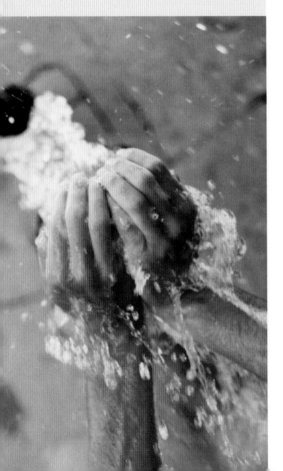

balancing body & mind

A successful detox programme depends on looking after your body and your mind as well as following an elimination diet. Taking good care of yourself is a necessity, not a luxury, because your physical well-being is intimately connected with the health of your mind and spirit. Exercise and beauty programmes complement the detox process because they promote circulation, sweating, deep breathing and flexibility. On an emotional level, they help to foster the sense of restoration and renewal.

Detox your body

This chapter shows you how to enhance your vitality through a daily body care routine which you can easily carry out at home. Specific body treatments, from home spa therapies and natural hair and skin products to foot massage and aromatherapy, will leave you feeling pampered and nurtured, as well as significantly improving the appearance of your skin and the efficiency of your body's elimination processes.

Regular exercise is essential, not just for detoxing but for a happy, healthy life. Apart from stimulating sweating, improving general metabolism and overall detoxification, exercise increases your self-esteem, reduces stress and makes your body work more efficiently. If exercise is something you normally avoid, read this chapter to find out why it is so important. There are also tips on how to get started and how to make exercise a pleasure rather than a chore. Exercise increases the production of free radicals (see page 9) in your body, so it must be accompanied by drinking sufficient fluids and the intake of antioxidant foods or supplements.

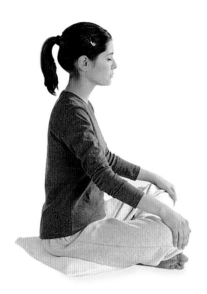

Your mind and body are thought to strive naturally towards equilibrium, or homeostasis, the maintenance of which is the key to good health. Balance is maintained by looking after the mind as well as the body. Optimum health depends on having a healthy diet, fresh air, exercise, sufficient rest and sleep, relaxation, managed stress levels, a clean environment and a positive mental attitude.

Detox your mind

This chapter also explores some of the various complementary therapies that abound to help promote good health and well-being, primarily through reducing stress levels. Stress has disastrous effects on your health – it affects how your body works and causes the production of harmful toxins. You will be shown how to reduce stress, detox your mind and restore your inner harmony through a series of simple exercises using tools such as meditation and visualization. Resting, relaxation and recharging are also important for detoxing. Relaxation exercises help your body rebalance and prevent negative thoughts from interfering with the body's natural processes.

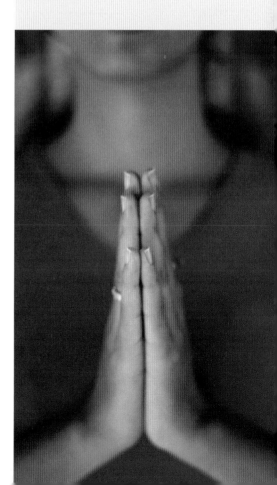

Mix 1 tbsp of honey with 2 tbsp finely ground almonds and ½ tsp lemon juice. Rub gently on to face and rinse off with warm water.

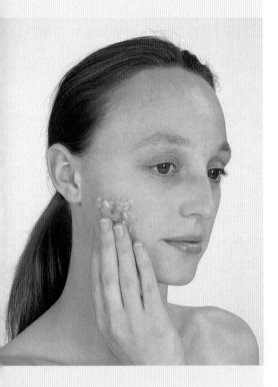

basic body detox

A daily and weekly body care routine, which you can easily carry out at home, will help improve the appearance of your skin and increase the elimination of toxins. It will also enhance your vitality and may help relieve digestive complaints. For extra pampering, treat yourself to at least one professional body treatment while detoxing.

SKIN BRUSHING

You lose about about 0.5 kg (1 lb) of waste products through the pores each day, so it makes sense to look after your skin. Brushing helps your skin 'breathe' efficiently by clearing the pores, and improves its appearance. It also boosts blood and lymph circulation, leading to more efficient excretion of waste materials in the cells and helping to relieve water retention.

How to brush your skin

Use a long-handled, natural bristle brush, or a loofah or a dry flannel. Do not wet or moisturize your skin and avoid brushing the face – the skin here is very delicate. Strokes should be long and firm, and towards your heart. Spend about 5 minutes a day dry-brushing your skin, following the sequence below. Your skin will tingle and you should feel quite warm afterwards because you have stimulated your circulation.

1   Start at your feet and work up your body. Brush both sides of your feet and up your legs.

2   Brush towards the heart and over the breast. Brush the stomach in

gentle, circular strokes in a clockwise direction. This follows the flow of your intestine.

3 Raise each arm in turn and brush from the hand to the armpit.

4 Brush from the buttocks up the back to the neck.

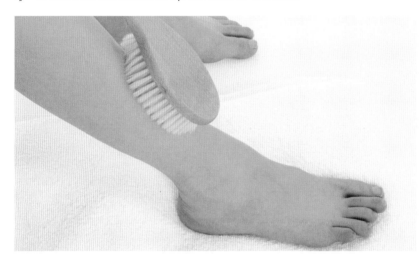

DAILY SHOWER OR BATH

Water can alter the body's blood flow and this can be manipulated by changing the water temperature. Hot water is relaxing. It dilates blood vessels, reducing blood pressure and increasing blood flow to the skin and muscles. The improved circulation helps remove waste products from the body and sends more oxygen and nutrients to the tissues to repair damage. Cold water is stimulating. It makes surface blood vessels constrict, restricting blood flow and sending blood towards the internal organs, helping them to function more efficiently. Having a warm bath or shower followed by a blast of cold water will do wonders for your circulation and skin.

EXFOLIATING BODY SCRUB

You can buy a ready-made scrub or make your own at home. The salt is the exfoliant, the oil or yogurt and honey moisturize the skin, and the essential oil helps to clear the body of toxins. Mix all the ingredients together in a bowl to make a runny paste.

1 tbsp sea salt

2 tbsp oil (olive, sunflower, etc.)
    or yogurt

1 tbsp thick honey

2–3 drops of sweet marjoram, rose,
    sweet fennel or juniper oil

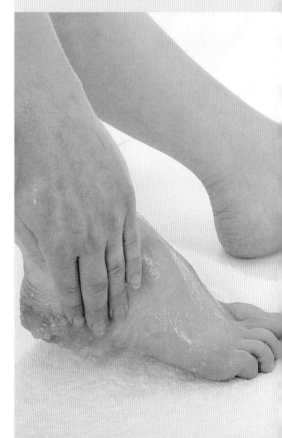

OILS FOR
FACE STEAMING

Dry skin Atlas cedarwood, geranium, neroli, rose, sandalwood

Sensitive skin Jasmine, lavender, Roman chamomile, rosewood

Oily skin Grapefruit, lemongrass, patchouli, sweet basil

Mature skin and wrinkles Clary sage, geranium, jasmine, lavender, rose, ylang-ylang

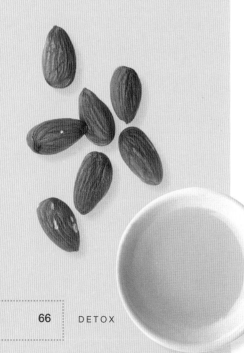

EXFOLIATION

Exfoliation gently removes dead skin cells and should be done at least once a week. You can use the exfoliating scrub (see page 64) or fill an old sock with oatmeal and swish it in your bathwater. Once the oatmeal has softened, scrub your body with it. For a very gentle exfoliant, add 125 ml (4 fl oz) cider apple vinegar to a lukewarm bath.

How to exfoliate

1   Relax in a warm bath for at least 10 minutes.
2   Lift each limb out of the water and rub your exfoliating scrub in firm circles all over your body, paying particular attention to areas of hard skin (e.g. the heels). Kneel up and exfoliate your buttocks and back.
3   Get out of the bath, gently pat yourself dry with a clean towel and apply a thick moisturizer or body oil.

OILS AND EMOLLIENTS

After bathing or showering you should always use oil or a good moisturizer to help your skin retain moisture. Essential oils, always used in a suitable carrier oil (see page 71), help your skin to eliminate impurities as well as keeping it soft. Rub olive oil into patches of eczema, dandruff and psoriasis both to reduce itching and also to promote healing.

EPSOM SALTS BATHS

As part of your body detox regime, try having an Epsom salts bath every 5 days, unless your skin is cut or grazed or you have a skin condition, in which case this type of bath should be avoided. Epsom salts are pure magnesium, which the body needs to help maintain healthy tissues, and it draws off toxins and improves circulation. Pour about 1 kg (2.2 lb) Epsom salts into bath water and stir until dissolved. Relax in the bath for 5 minutes, then massage your skin with a massage mitt or flannel.

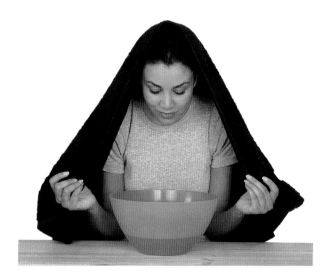

FACIALS

Deep-clean your face once a week to remove impurities from skin pores. Start off by cleaning your face using your normal cleanser. Next, fill a bowl with very hot water and then add a few drops of an essential oil appropriate for your skin type (see box opposite). Lean over the bowl, with your head covered by a towel and your eyes closed for 10 minutes. Use cotton wool to wipe your face clean, then soak your face using a warm, moist cloth. Apply a commercial skin mask suitable for your skin type, or you could make your own from the recipes provided (see box), and leave it on for 15 minutes. Gently remove the face mask using a cool, wet cloth. Finally, apply a moisturizer.

Dry skin Take 1 tbsp of porridge oats and rub well between your fingers. Steep in a cup of boiling water for 20 minutes. Strain, then mix the oats with 1 tbsp honey, 1 egg yolk and 1 tbsp natural yogurt. Apply to the skin with cotton wool and leave on for 15 minutes.

Sensitive skin Mix 1 tsp aloe vera gel (available from chemists or healthfood stores) with 1 tbsp natural yogurt. Apply and leave for 15 minutes.

Oily skin Mix 1 tbsp dry fuller's earth (available from healthfood shops or chemists) with 1 egg yolk, $\frac{1}{4}$ mashed avocado and a little witch hazel to create a smooth mixture. Apply to the skin and leave on for 15 minutes.

Mature skin Mash a ripe avocado with a little olive oil and apply to the skin. Leave on for 15 minutes.

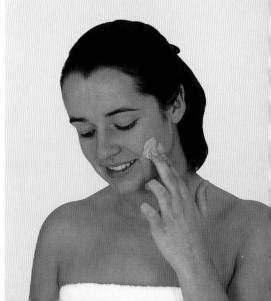

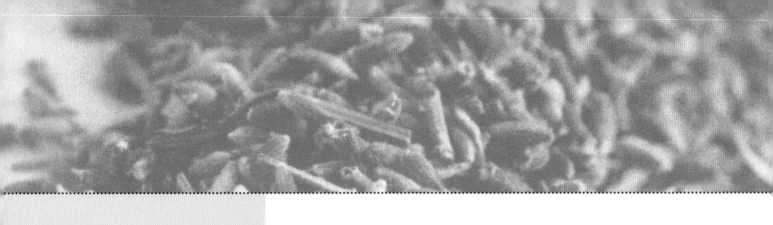

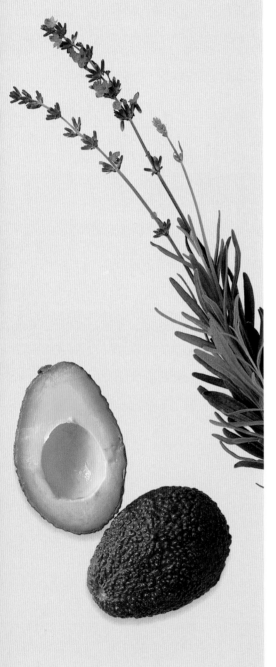

SCALP MASSAGE

A scalp massage and hair mask can help ensure glossy, healthy hair. Do this at least once a week if you can. Massage essential oils into your hair to regulate hair-oil production and improve the condition of your scalp. Use 1 tbsp of carrier oil (see page 71) and 2 drops of essential oil. For greasy hair, choose from clary sage, geranium, lemon, lavender, tea tree, cypress and rosemary; for dry hair, choose from Roman chamomile (blond hair only), lavender and rosemary; and for dandruff, choose from tea tree, juniper, lemon, lavender and sandalwood.

Massage the oil into the scalp using your fingertips, leave for half an hour then rinse off. Towel hair dry then follow with the antioxidant fruit smoothie hair mask.

Fruit smoothie hair mask

In a food processor or blender, mix ½ banana, ¼ melon, ¼ avocado, 1 tbsp olive oil and 1 tbsp yogurt. Work the mixture into the roots of your hair then coat all the remaining hair. Wrap your head in clingfilm and allow to penetrate for 15 minutes. Rinse your hair well in warm water then lightly shampoo and rinse again, and leave to dry naturally.

HAND AND FOOT CARE

These simple techniques use elements of massage (see page 70) and reflexology (see page 74) to help remove blockages and eliminate toxins. Do this once a week.

Hand massage

Gently stroke the front and back of each hand to relax and warm it. Mix 1 tbsp sea salt with 2 tsp olive oil and 3–4 drops lavender essential oil. Scoop into your hands and rub your hands together. Cover the entire hand and wrist area and leave for 1 minute. Rinse in warm water. Use your thumb to stroke from the knuckle of your little finger down the tendon towards the wrist. Repeat for each finger. Gently grip a finger with the knuckles of the first two fingers of the other hand. Slide down the finger to the fingertip, pulling with a corkscrew-like motion. Repeat twice on each finger and thumb. Use the opposite thumb to massage across the palm several times. Apply knuckle pressures to the palm, then gently stroke it. Repeat the whole sequence on the other hand.

Foot massage

Fill a large bowl with warm water and then soak your feet for 10 minutes. Using a pumice stone, remove dead skin on the heels and sides. Apply some massage oil to your hands. Using quite firm pressure, rub your hands all over your foot and up over your ankle. Using your thumbs, massage the entire surface of your foot in tiny, deep circles. Use the same stroke on the underside of your foot. If you touch an area of the foot that is sore, hold the point with your thumb until the discomfort lessens. Then massage up the inside edge of the foot, from the heel to the tip of the big toe. Wiggle your toes then pull on each toe from the tip. Once you have finished the sequence, repeat it for the other foot.

COLONIC IRRIGATION

Although not part of mainstream detox, some people visit a trained professional for some sessions of colonic irrigation after a couple of weeks of detoxing. The aim is to remove impacted faeces from the colon, ensuring that the toxins in it are not reabsorbed. You will be asked to lie face down with your lower body covered, before filtered water is gently pumped into the rectum to soften and flush away built-up toxins and waste. The colon is worked on in stages: water is pumped in and flushed out each time until the whole area is treated.

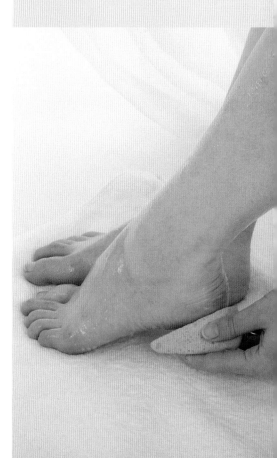

massage

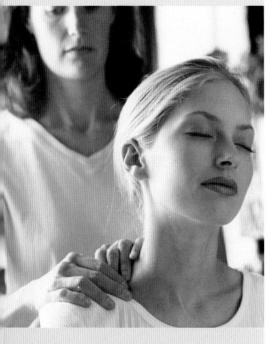

Therapeutic massage is an ancient technique used to promote general well-being and enhance self-esteem, while boosting the circulatory and lymphatic systems and reducing tension. It improves the supply of oxygen and nutrients to body tissues, enhances skin tone, and increases the elimination of chemical wastes from the body. At the same time it is an agreeable and soothing experience.

There are numerous kinds of massage, many of which have been incorporated into a variety of complementary therapies, but for detox purposes aromatherapy massage and therapeutic massage are the best. You can massage yourself, though it is not as relaxing as being massaged by somebody else.

During a full body massage, which lasts about an hour, the practitioner will use a light vegetable oil or talcum powder to enable their hands to glide over the skin. Most strokes are carried out slowly and rhythmically towards the heart to help increase the blood and lymph circulation.

Basic techniques

Effleurage (stroking) is a gentle action for all parts of the body to warm and relax the muscles and aid circulation. Kneading techniques stretch and tone muscles. Pétrissage is similar to kneading in effect, but involves just using the thumbs and fingertips. Wringing, using the whole hand, is used on larger areas of the body. Percussion techniques, including tapotement, involve hacking with the sides of the hands to deliver short, sharp taps on the body.

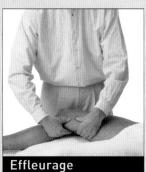

Effleurage

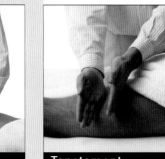

Tapotement

aromatherapy

Aromatherapy uses aromatic essential oils extracted from herbs, flowers, fruits and trees. The oils are thought to penetrate the skin and travel through the body via the bloodstream and lymph vessels. The oils are extremely potent and should not be applied directly to the skin or taken internally, and many oils are not suitable for use during pregnancy.

Essential oils are diluted in a vegetable-based carrier oil such as almond or grapeseed oil, or blended in a lotion or cream. A normal dilution is 6 drops of essential oil (or a combination of up to three different oils) per 20 ml (4 tsp) of carrier oil, which is sufficient for a full body massage.

Basic techniques

- **Massage** Diluted as above
- **Bathing** Add to bathwater, breaking up the oil on the surface to prevent it from burning the skin
- **Steam inhalation** Add 2–3 drops to a bowl of steaming hot water, lean your face over the bowl, drape a towel over your head and breathe in the steam for a few minutes

Ten key oils for body detox

Basil, fennel, juniper, lemon, mandarin, marjoram, peppermint, pine, rose, rosemary

Ten key oils for mind detox

Atlas cedarwood, chamomile, eucalyptus, geranium, jasmine, lavender, lemon balm, lime, rose, ylang-ylang

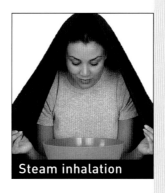

Steam inhalation

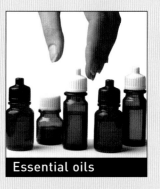

Essential oils

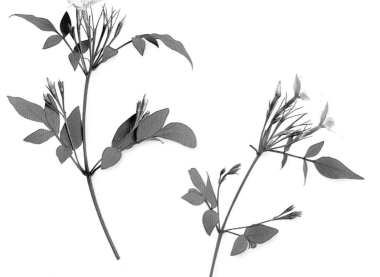

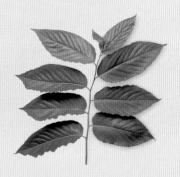

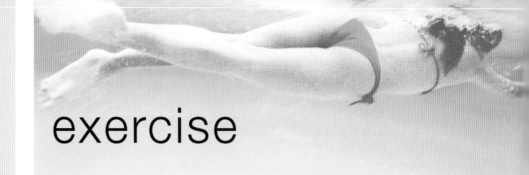

exercise

CONSULT YOUR DOCTOR

You should consult your doctor if you have not exercised regularly for several years or if you are overweight or have a medical condition. Your doctor may recommend certain types of exercise that are more appropriate for you.

Exercise helps your body eliminate toxins and is an essential part of any detox regime. Regular gentle exercise also builds up your stamina, flexibility and strength, and is invaluable in maintaining a healthy body, mind and spirit. Repetitive exercise such as swimming, walking or running is also a golden opportunity for you to enjoy self-reflection, mental relaxation and meditation.

Key benefits of exercise

- Muscular movement enables your body's systems to work more efficiently, removing toxins
- Increases muscle strength, which can help to prevent back pain
- Makes your body more efficient at using oxygen
- Promotes deep breathing, which is key to relaxation
- Makes you physically tired and aids sleep
- Causes the release of the body's natural painkillers, endorphins, which reduce anxiety and leave you feeling relaxed and in a better mood
- Releases adrenalin, thus reducing stress
- Improves self-esteem
- Strengthens the heart and helps reduce blood pressure
- Helps control cholesterol and burns fat
- Improves circulation
- Speeds up metabolism
- Increases your body's ability to fight off infection
- Improves joint mobility and stability, which can help to keep you active and independent in later life

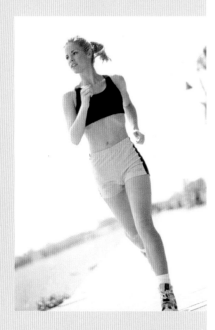

- Helps keep bones strong and healthy
- Meditative exercise such as t'ai chi help you focus your mind and improve coordination

Ways of getting started

You don't have to join a gym to start to get fit. There are many things you can do that you may not have considered to be exercise that are easily incorporated into your life: walk up the stairs instead of taking the lift, walk or cycle to work, take the dog for regular walks, take the children to play in the park at the weekend and join in (and this will benefit the whole family, not just yourself), or simply put on some music and dance around the living room.

To start exercising, aim to do 15–20 minutes at least three times a week. Follow an exercise routine you enjoy, such as swimming, walking or cycling, because you are much more likely to stick to it. The aim is to inspire you to incorporate exercise into your daily routine long after you have finished the detox programme. As your body gets stronger you should increase the length and intensity of the exercise, but always be aware of how your body is feeling during and after exercise. If you feel exhausted, take more rest until your vitality increases. Build up gradually, especially if you have not exercised for a while.

Once you have built up your strength and restored your energy levels you can move on to regular cardiovascular exercise. This enhances detoxing and increases the oxygen uptake in your body. Cycling, running, swimming, tennis, yoga and aerobics are all suitable. Aim to exercise for at least half an hour five times a week.

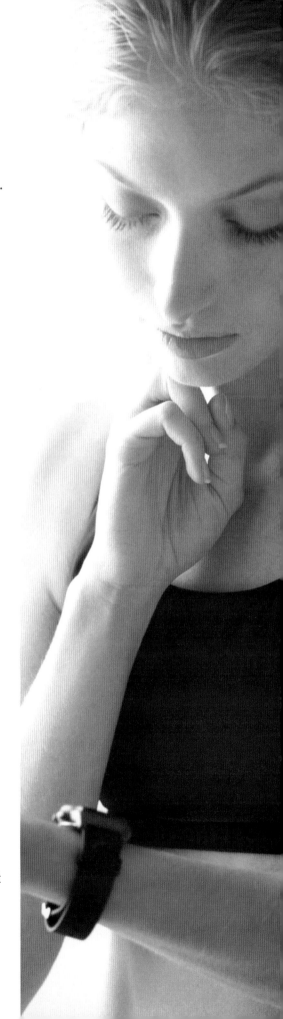

reflexology

Hand and foot massage have long been used to promote relaxation and improve health. Practitioners of reflexology believe that the feet and hands are mirrors of the whole body and that pressure placed on specific reflex points on them can be used to treat the corresponding areas of the body, promoting well-being and stimulating the body's natural healing powers. Reflexology is a good complementary therapy for detoxing the body and the mind. Massaging the feet allows blood to circulate more freely, distributing oxygen and nutrients through the body and removing waste products.

Reflexology can help your body detox by encouraging the organs of elimination to work well. Stimulating the reflex points is thought to help eliminate waste products, which are felt as tender granular or crystalline deposits in the feet or hands. The aim is to break down these deposits and improve the blood supply to flush away toxins. Specific reflex points to work on while detoxing include the spleen/pancreas, stomach, adrenal glands, colon, liver, gallbladder and kidneys.

Basic techniques

Practitioners usually work with the feet because they are more sensitive. The practitioner gives an initial massage to relax the feet and then massages the whole of each foot to stimulate the reflex points. Extra massage is given to break down crystalline deposits and free energy flow. The practitioner will use the pad of the thumb to move over the skin, applying and releasing pressure before creeping along slightly and repeating the action. You can practise reflexology on your own hands or feet, though you will benefit more from a professional treatment.

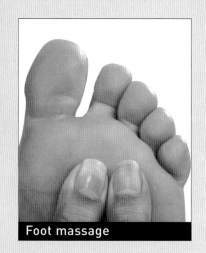
Foot massage

yoga

Practised for thousands of years, yoga was originally developed as a system of mental and physical training in preparation for spiritual growth. There are many types of yoga, all of which incorporate various asanas (postures) and breathing techniques. Yoga enables you to cultivate a fit and flexible body as well as a balanced mind and emotions.

Various yoga postures can be extremely helpful for detoxing because they stimulate the digestion and lymphatic system. Others improve circulation and increase the supply of oxygen. Everyone, regardless of age or fitness level, can benefit from yoga.

Basic techniques

It is very important to join a yoga class or take lessons from a qualified practitioner. After guiding you through some gentle warm-up exercises, your teacher will show you the correct way to perform yoga postures, which you then practise with the rest of the class, followed by a period of relaxation.

When practising yoga by yourself you should progress gradually and never force your body into postures before you are ready. Aim to practise for at least 20 minutes daily to increase your energy and stamina, tone muscles, improve digestion, help you deal with stress and improve concentration. Allow three hours after a meal before exercising. Seek medical advice before doing upside-down poses such as shoulderstands if you have any physical problems affecting your heart, neck, blood pressure, ears or eyes.

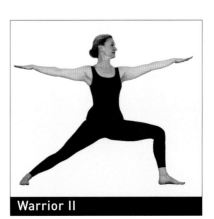

Warrior II

Sitting stretch

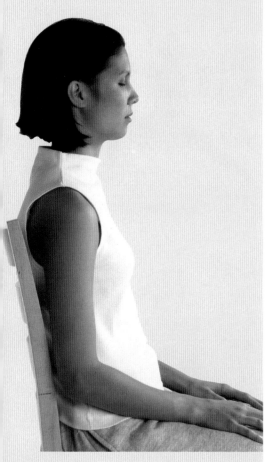

breathing & relaxation

Controlled breathing and simple muscle-relaxation techniques can be practised to reduce the physical and mental effects of stress, which can cause the build-up of unwanted toxins in your body. If you find it difficult to begin a breathing and relaxation programme on your own, try consulting a practitioner who can talk you through various techniques.

BREATHING

Breathing is essential for life: as you breathe, oxygen is taken into the lungs and released into the bloodstream, where it fuels the production of energy that enables your body to function. If you are stressed, your breathing tends to be shallow, using only the top part of the lungs. There is a drop in levels of carbon dioxide, which is needed to maintain blood acidity, and harmful toxins are not breathed out. This affects the nerves and muscles and may result in tiredness, palpitations and panic attacks. If you learn to breathe properly you can alleviate these conditions and you will also benefit from a lower heart rate, reduced blood pressure and lower levels of stress hormones.

How to breathe deeply

If you find your breathing is too fast or too shallow, the following exercise – known as abdominal breathing – will help you breathe more deeply. It uses the diaphragm, the sheet of muscle forming the top of the abdomen, to enable the lungs to inflate and deflate with minimal effort.

1   Sit in a comfortable position. Place one hand on your chest and the
    other over your diaphragm just below the breastbone. Breathe in

slowly through your nose, and try to breathe so that the hand on your chest remains relatively still.

2   Hold the breath for a few seconds then breathe out slowly through your nose. Release as much air as possible.

3   Repeat three or four times. Throughout the exercise, try to concentrate solely on your breathing.

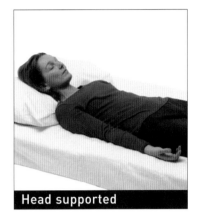
Head supported

RELAXATION

When your body and mind are under pressure, your muscles become constricted. This restricts the blood supply, making it harder for the body to eliminate toxins, and can dramatically affect the way your body functions. The following technique will help you to relax all the major muscle groups.

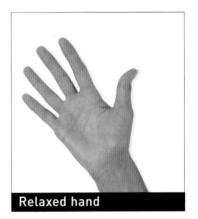
Relaxed hand

1   Lie down with a pillow under your head for support. Close your eyes and focus on breathing slowly.

2   Tense the muscle in your right foot, hold for a few seconds then release. Tense and release the calf, then the thigh muscles. Repeat with the left foot and leg.

3   Tense and release the muscles in your right hand and arm, then the left.

4   Tense and release each buttock, then the stomach muscles.

5   Lift your shoulders up to your ears, hold for a few seconds, then lower. Repeat three times. Rock your head gently from side to side.

6   Yawn, then pout. Frown, wrinkle your nose and let go. Raise your eyebrows then relax your face muscles.

7   Focus on your breathing again. Wiggle your fingers and toes, bend your knees and roll on to your side. Get up slowly.

meditation & visualization

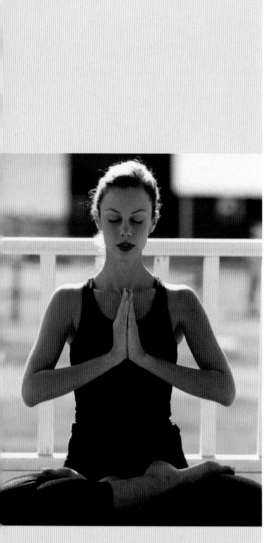

Meditation and visualization help you achieve and maintain inner harmony; they are also important for detoxing because they reduce stress levels. If stress persists, the stress hormones adrenalin and cortisol interfere with the functioning of the circulatory and immune systems, making it harder for the body to detoxify properly. If you are not used to meditating or visualization you may find them quite hard to do at first, but regular practice will soon lead to their becoming second nature. As you become more experienced in controlling your mind you may be able to switch to a relaxed state despite the distractions of the bustle of life around you.

Key principles

A practitioner can show you how to achieve a meditative state, but you can teach yourself if you are sufficiently disciplined. In order to meditate successfully there are a few basic requirements:

- A quiet place where you will not be disturbed
- Regular practice, preferably at the same time each day
- An empty stomach
- A comfortable position
- A focus for the mind to help you withdraw from your surroundings: this can be an object such as a plant, candle or picture; a mantra (a word or phrase repeated continually, either silently or aloud); rhythmically passing a rosary or worry beads through your fingers; focusing on your breathing; or repetitive, rhythmic exercise such as swimming or t'ai chi

Basic meditation

1　Sit up in a comfortable position with your spine straight. Keep your eyes open or closed, depending on the method of meditation you are using. Rest your hands in your lap.

2　Breathe slowly and rhythmically, and try to stay as still as possible.

3　Focus on the object of your meditation and allow your attention to be passive. If your mind starts to wander, acknowledge what is happening then return to your focus.

4　Continue for as long as is comfortable – for a few minutes to start with, building up to 20 minutes a day.

5　When you are ready, open your eyes, then take a minute to become fully aware of your surroundings.

VISUALIZATION

This is a technique that harnesses the imagination to create positive mental images to deal with stress and illness. Through imagination, you can use positive thinking to stimulate the body's natural healing abilities.

Basic visualization

Choose a quiet place where you won't be disturbed. Breathe slowly and relax. Focus on your chosen mental image. To combat stress, visualize a calm, beautiful scene and picture yourself there. Repeat positive affirmations as you do this, such as 'I am relaxed and happy'. To facilitate detoxing, you can visualize how clean you will be when you have finished the programme, and you can affirm your ability to follow the programme successfully. Repeat the exercise at least once more during the day.

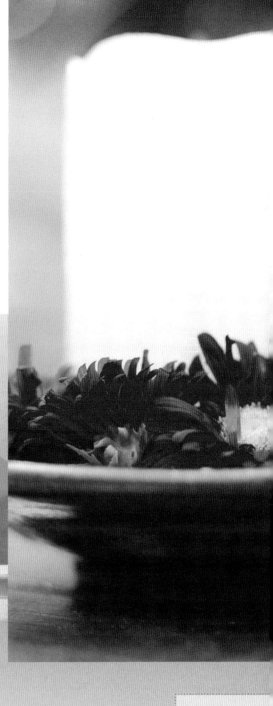

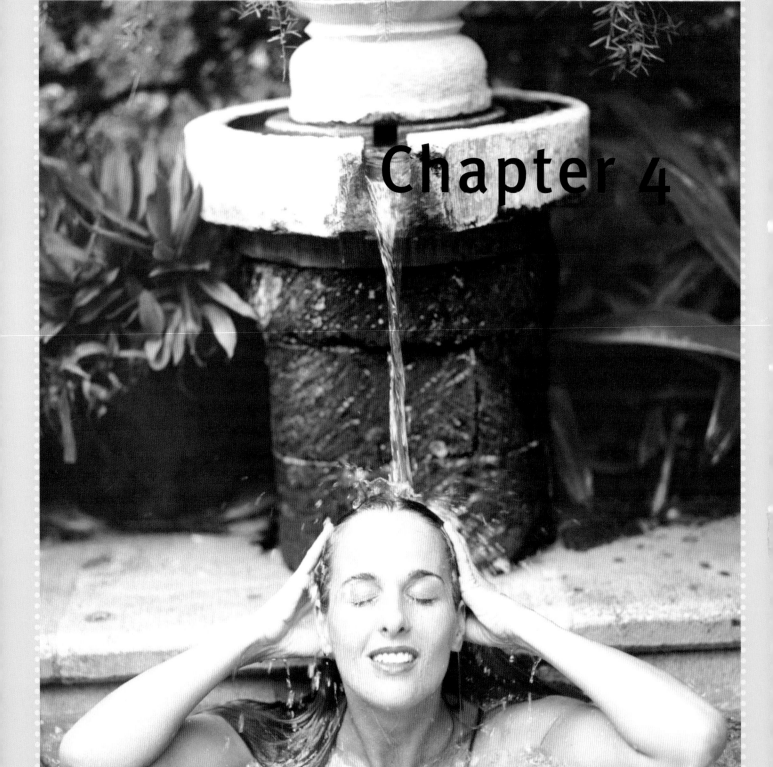

Chapter 4

DETOX IN
A WEEKEND

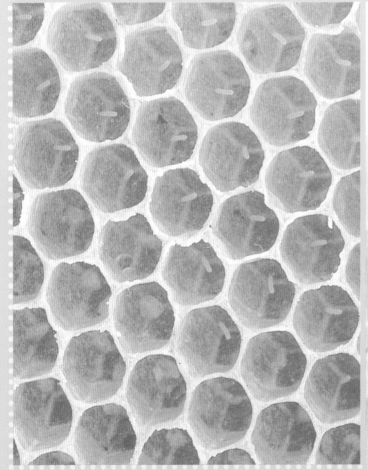

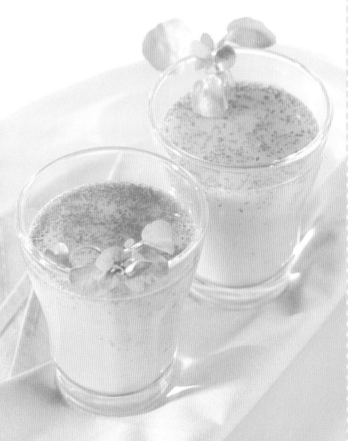

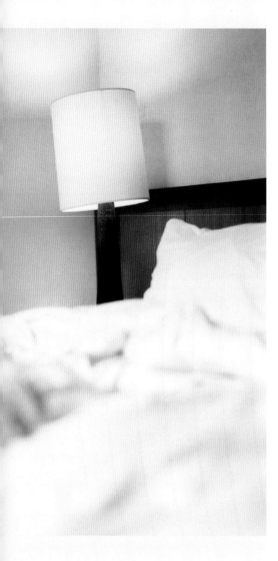

home health farm

Following a short detox programme will give your body a break from its toxic load and leave you feeling refreshed, invigorated and ready for action. It includes all the elements of detoxing to enable your body to get rid of waste products more effectively and improve your underlying health. It's also all about pampering yourself from top to toe. A trip to a health farm can be an expensive luxury, but with a little planning you can easily create your own health farm at home where you can detox for the weekend.

What's in the programme

The food detox element is a programme of light eating that incorporates juices to stimulate the cleansing organs of the body, as well as giving your digestive system a rest. Other elements include various treatments, such as aromatherapy, massage and body scrubs, and they are intended to help the detox process as well as making you feel and look good. You will also need to exercise to make your body function more efficiently and to help the elimination process. The spiritual element incorporates meditation and visualization to help you detox your mind and induce inner harmony.

Environment

Make sure your house is clean and tidy – or at least the rooms you will be using – so that you are not distracted by the need to do housework. Your bedsheets should be clean and fresh, as should your nightwear/ leisurewear and dressing gown. Turn the heating up a notch as you will be sitting around in loose clothing.

Equipment

- Selection of reading material (none of it should be work-related)
- Notepad or diary and something to write with
- Art materials: raid your children's supplies for paper, pencils or crayons, paints or modelling clay, or treat yourself to a cheap kit
- Rug or duvet
- Lots of pillows
- Essential oils for relaxation – lavender, rose or jasmine. Dilute 6 drops of essential oil per 20 ml (4 tsp) of carrier oil such as almond or grapeseed oil
- Candles
- Music to relax to or a relaxation tape. Classical music or nature sounds work well – visit the local library if you don't have anything suitable and borrow some tapes or CDs for the weekend

Food

- Variety of fresh fruit and vegetables
- Unwaxed lemons
- Herbal teas and filtered or bottled water
- Olive oil
- Selection of nuts and seeds
- Goat's or ewe's milk yogurt
- Brown rice
- Fresh herbs

Choose from the shopping list on pages 24-25 to plan your menu and buy produce as required.

CREATING A HOME SPA

When it comes to the bathroom, we want to be pampered as if we're at an expensive spa. Most of us can't install Japanese-style hot tubs, but it is possible to turn an ordinary bathroom into a luxurious sanctuary so that you can feel relaxed and rejuvenated.

- Have large, thick cotton bath towels and soft flannels available
- Install some aromatherapy candles – the soft glow will make you feel relaxed and the aroma will be calming
- Combine almond oil with a few drops of your favourite essential oil. Store in a decorative glass container and add to bathwater
- Have an exfoliating scrub, face mask, loofah and moisturizer available

You can make up your own menu
from the list of permitted foods on
pages 24-25, but some suggestions
are given below to help you get
going. Don't forget to drink at least
eight glasses of liquid a day to help
flush out toxins.

breakfast Fresh fruit or fruit
smoothie

mid-morning break A handful of
dried fruit and nuts or bunch of
grapes

lunch Grilled goat's cheese with
grilled vegetables, plus brown rice
and mixed leaf salad

afternoon snack Half an avocado, or
crudités with Hummus (see page 38),
or vegetable juice

dinner Grilled Vegetable Soup (see
page 40) followed by fresh fruit

detox schedule

This short programme is designed to be carried out over a weekend
because that's usually when most people can be free of work, but you can
do this during the week if more convenient. Plan in advance to make the
detox programme go as smoothly as possible. If you have a partner and/or
children, arrange for them to go away for the weekend. You don't have to
follow the timetables slavishly – they're designed to give you a rough idea
of how long each activity will take; do the programme at your own pace.

Before you start

In the two days leading up to your weekend detox, cut down on tea and
coffee, red meat, processed foods and alcohol. This will help reduce
withdrawal symptoms, but be prepared to feel headachy, hungry and
lethargic on the Saturday.

What to avoid

As well as following the weekend detox programme as closely as possible,
a few things should be eliminated to make it most effective. Avoid coffee,
alcohol, cigarettes and non-essential drugs. Avoid salt and oil, and use
fresh herbs and lemon or lime juice to dress and season your food.
The meal suggestions given do not specify quantities but, because you
want to give your digestive system a rest, it's best not to eat too much.
If you feel hungry, try a piece of fresh fruit or raw vegetable.

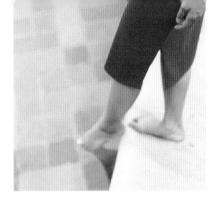

friday evening

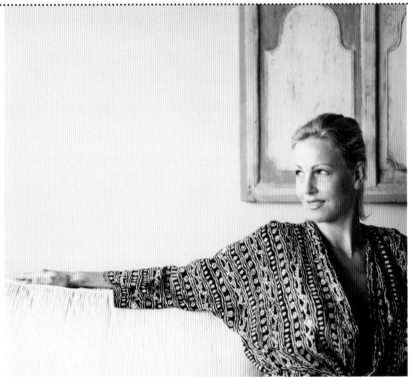

Ease yourself into the detox by getting everything ready in advance. Change into comfortable clothes and have a light supper of grilled fish and salad. Turn your bathroom into a home spa (see page 83), put the answering machine on and get ready to revitalize yourself.

Winding down

At about 8.30 p.m., fill the bath with very hot water and add a few drops of essential oil. Leave for 10 minutes to heat up the tub and let the oils disperse. Make yourself a cup of herbal tea to sip while bathing, light the candles and put on some relaxing music. Immerse yourself in the bath, lie back and relax. Afterwards, get out slowly and pat yourself dry. You should be feeling sleepy, so put on your nightclothes and head for bed.

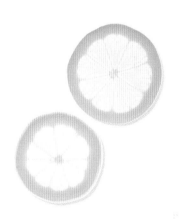

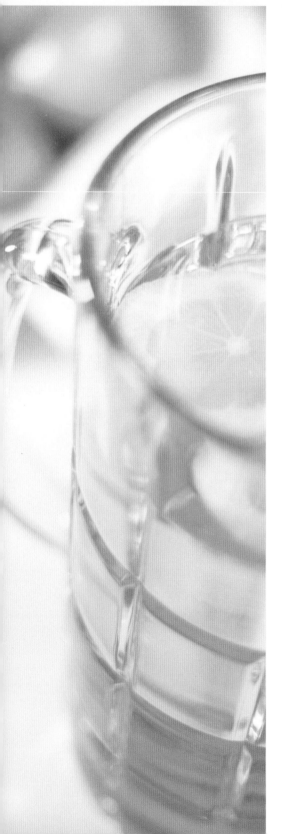

saturday

MORNING PROGRAMME

Have a lie-in when you wake up, then drink a glass of hot water and lemon juice. Follow this with a dry skin brushing session (see page 64), then take a hot shower or bath, followed by a blast of cold water. Dress in loose clothes, and eat a light breakfast. Write down in your diary or notepad all that is going through your mind. If you are worried, you should be able to see the problems and put them into perspective. If you are happy, writing down your thoughts will help to prolong your mood. Then practise the exercises for deep breathing and muscle relaxation on pages 76–77. Before lunch, relax by reading, then meditate (see pages 78–79).

AFTERNOON PROGRAMME

Take a long walk somewhere where you can appreciate nature and get plenty of fresh air. You mustn't drive to get there because this will raise your stress levels again; if there is nowhere pleasant nearby, take a bus or train to your chosen destination. After your walk, give yourself a foot massage (see page 69), then it's time for a home beauty session. Have a deep-cleaning facial (see page 67), then massage your scalp with a dilution of lavender oil or apply the fruit smoothie hair mask (see page 68). Follow this by relaxing in the living room, reading or watching a film.

EVENING PROGRAMME

Wind down for the evening with a light supper that your body can digest easily. Then have another relaxation session – reading, writing, listening to music. Light some candles and think positive thoughts. End the evening with a hand massage (see page 69), then go to bed.

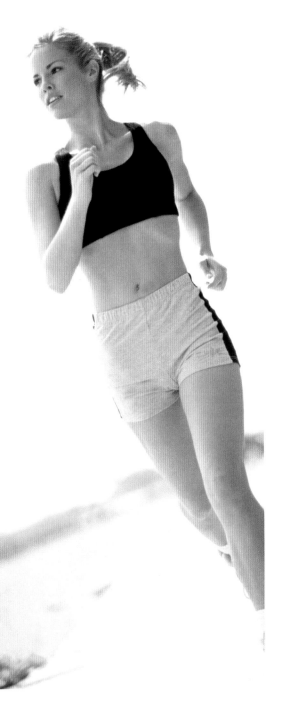

PLAN YOUR DAY AHEAD

9:30am   lemon juice & hot water

9:45am   dry skin brush & shower

10:00am   breakfast

10:15am   rest & relaxation

11:30am   mid-morning break

12:00pm   rest & meditation

1:00pm   lunch

2:00pm   long walk

4:00pm   afternoon snack

4:15pm   home beauty salon

5:30pm   relaxation

7:00pm   supper

8:00pm   relaxation & hand massage

10:00pm   bed

sunday

You need to ease back into eating after finishing the programme. Have non-dairy (i.e. soya, ewe's milk or goat's milk) yogurt with muesli and fresh fruit for breakfast (see pages 36-37); add a little protein in the form of grilled or poached lean meat or fish later in the day. Try not to slip back completely into your old bad habits, but don't restrict your diet so much that you feel bored or resentful. Indulge yourself when socially necessary and at other times keep yourself well-nourished by maintaining a high intake of fresh fruit and vegetables.

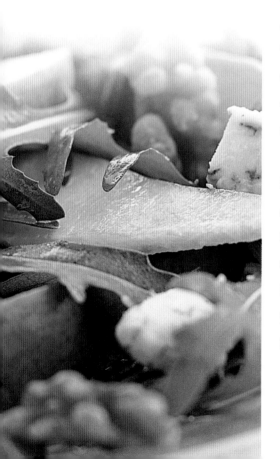

MORNING PROGRAMME

Start the day with a glass of hot water with a squeeze of lemon in it. Have a light breakfast, then dry brush your skin and get dressed in loose, comfortable clothing. Follow this with a moderate workout: do a few stretches to loosen and warm up your muscles, then go for a brisk walk around the block, dig over a flowerbed or mow the lawn, or put some music on and dance around the living room – anything that will make you sweat and your heart work faster. Then it's time to use your home spa to speed up the detox process. Run a hot bath and apply an Exfoliating Scrub (see page 65). Then retire to the living room for breathing and relaxation exercises (see pages 76–77) before lunch.

AFTERNOON PROGRAMME

Activities such as painting, drawing or moulding clay are excellent outlets for your emotions and can be deeply relaxing. Talent is not at stake – you do not have to produce a fantastic work of art. Let yourself become aware of the different textures and aromas of the art materials you are using and enjoy the experience. Alternatively, you could make a trip to an art gallery.

EVENING PROGRAMME

As you near the end of the weekend detox you are likely to find that your thoughts are far less cluttered or confused. This is the time to write a list or series of steps for achievable goals after detox in different areas of your life – relationships, work, financial matters, lifestyle, for example – and set yourself realistic timetables. Follow this with a light supper and then relax in front of the TV or with a good book, before retiring to bed.

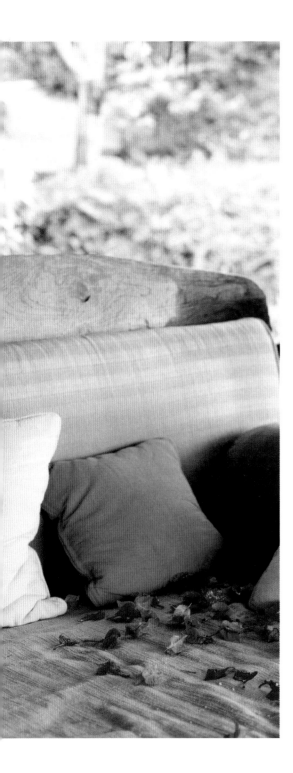

PLAN YOUR DAY AHEAD

9:00am   lemon juice & hot water

9:30am   breakfast

9:45am   skin brushing

10:00am   active session

10:30am   mid-morning break

11:00am   home spa treatment

12:00pm   deep breathing & relaxation

1:00pm   lunch

1:30pm   creative relaxation

3:00pm   afternoon snack

3:15pm   visualization & rest

4:30pm   planning session

6:30pm   light supper

10:00pm   bed

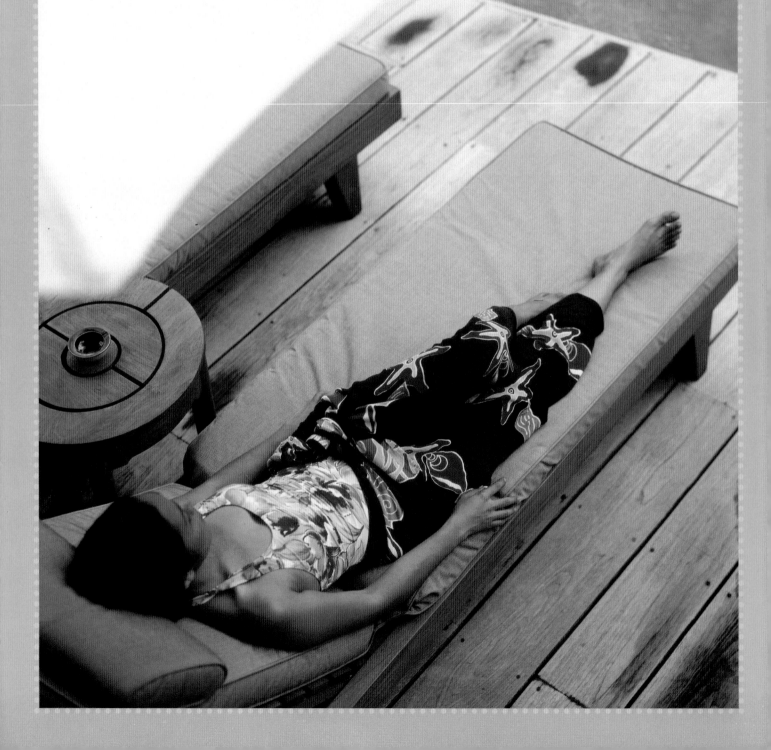

Chapter 5

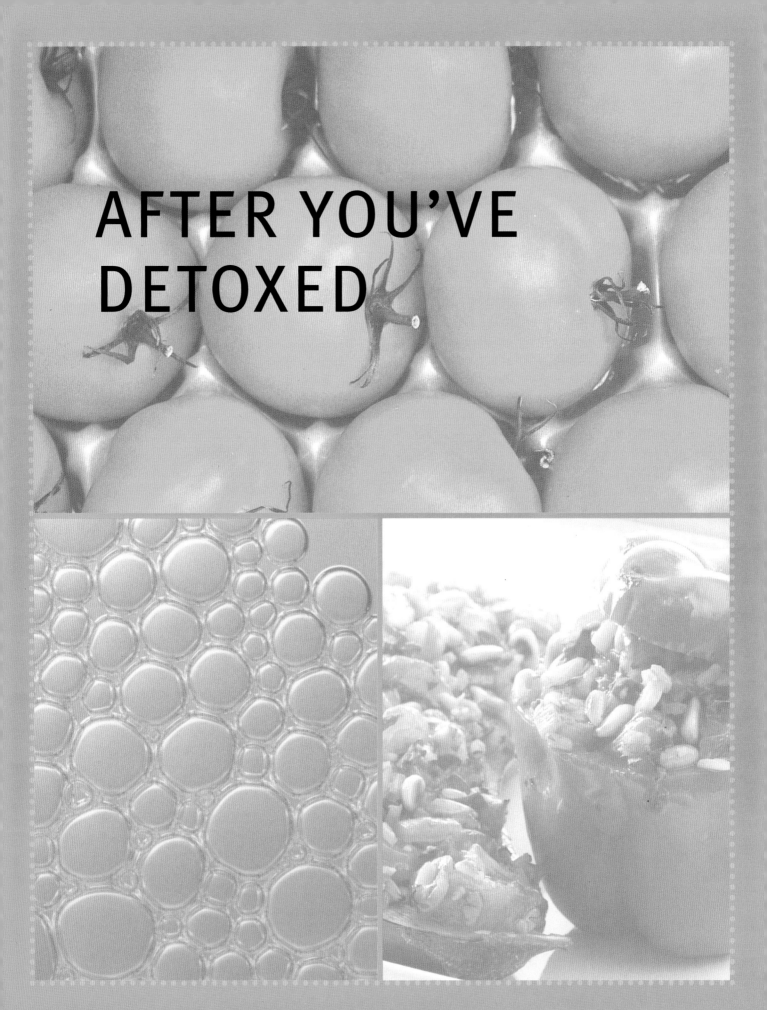

AFTER YOU'VE DETOXED

- Eat oily fish at least twice a week for the essential fatty acids (EFAs) vital for good metabolism – if you can't stand fish, you can still get your EFAs from flax seeds (linseed) or by taking a supplement
- Soya products such as tofu, soya milk and yogurt are excellent sources of low-fat protein
- Live yogurt contains friendly bacteria to keep your intestines healthy
- Berry fruits such as grapes, blueberries, strawberries and raspberries contain large amounts of antioxidant nutrients

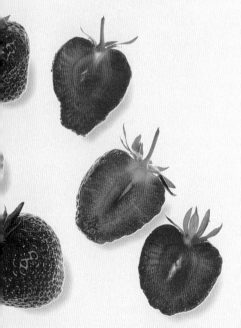

detox principles for life

Having completed the detox programme, you should be feeling a good deal healthier and more energetic than you did before. The idea from now on is to avoid a build-up of toxins in your body by sticking to healthy eating patterns. You should also keep up your exercise and relaxation routines, and continue to look after your body. If you can avoid a constant diet of junk food, alcohol and caffeine, and manage stress effectively, you shouldn't need a drastic detox regime in the future.

REINTRODUCING FOOD

When reintroducing food into your regular diet it is best to tackle one particular group at a time: this way you can work out if a particular type of food doesn't agree with you. Keeping a food diary is the best way of doing

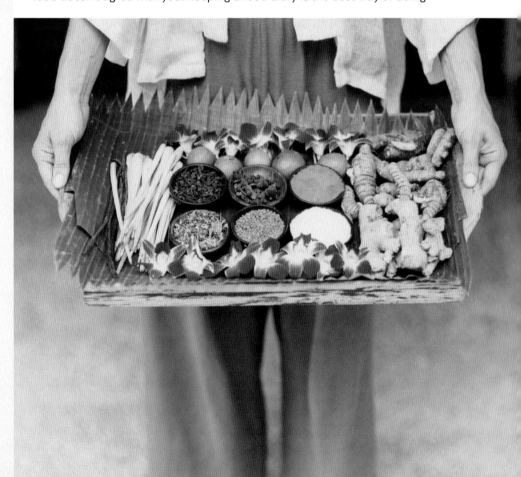

this. Note down what you have eaten and drunk, the approximate quantities and relevant details such as whether or not the product is organic, and any symptoms such as tiredness or bloating that you feel during the day. At the end of the week go through the diary and look for patterns. For example, you may notice that you feel tired or get headaches after eating pasta. If you think you may have a food intolerance it is important to consult a nutritionist for professional advice on how to modify your diet.

How to eat well for life

Once you have experienced the benefits of detoxing and become accustomed to a new way of eating, you can easily incorporate the main principles into your regular diet. Planning is key here.

Stock up Keep your larder stocked with ingredients that will enable you to prepare quick, healthy meals. Oatcakes, non-wheat pasta, lentils, brown rice, quinoa, tinned tomatoes, dried fruit, a selection of nuts and seeds, canned chickpeas and cannellini beans, and canned tuna in oil are all good standbys. In the freezer, keep a supply of frozen peas, sweetcorn and broad beans.

Plan ahead Plan your meals for the week and make a list before you go shopping, as this will help you avoid buying unhealthy food. Buy your fruit and vegetables loose rather than prepacked – the soft plastics they are wrapped in contain chemicals that are thought to disrupt hormones, your body's chemical messengers.

- Celery, cucumber and watermelon all help eliminate excess fluid
- Digestive system superfoods include papaya, pineapple, carrots, broccoli and cabbage, all packed with antioxidants and soluble fibre
- Eat a variety of different-coloured foods, because each colour contains different health-giving phytonutrients
- Drink at least 1.5 litres (3 pints) of fluid a day to flush out toxins

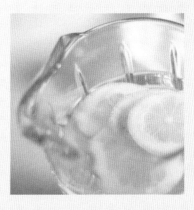

1 small banana, sliced

1 pot live low-fat yogurt

1 tsp honey

1 tsp sunflower seeds

1 tbsp muesli

Mix together all the ingredients and
eat. This breakfast will balance your
blood sugars and provide a sustained
release of energy. Banana
replenishes your potassium stocks,
crucial for maintaining fluid levels
and the correct balance of acid
to alkaline.

hangover detox

Most of us at one time or another drink more than we should. The most
common side effects of drinking too much are headaches, nausea and
tiredness, resulting from a combination of dehydration and inability of the
liver to flush out toxins quickly enough. This programme is designed to
help you overcome the side effects and help repair the internal and
external damage, but it doesn't mean you can drink to excess whenever
you feel like it. Drinking too much is very bad for your long-term health: if
you think you may have an addiction you should seek professional help.

BEFORE YOU START DRINKING
Top up with water

Drink at least 1.5 litres (3 pints) of water in each of the days leading up to
the big night out – this will make sure you are fully hydrated and help to
flush out toxins.

Eat something

Have a meal before you go out and don't drink on an empty stomach –
alcohol is very acidic.

Supplement

Take a B-complex vitamin and 1 g of vitamin C, both of which are used up
when alcohol is being broken down in the body.

WHILE YOU'RE DRINKING
Drink more slowly

Having a glass of water after every alcoholic drink is a useful technique.

Avoid bubbles

The bubbles in sparkling alcoholic drinks such as champagne or rum-and-
coke speed up alcohol absorption, making you drunk more quickly.

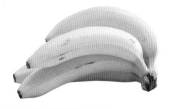

Drink according to your size and sex

Women are less able to break down alcohol than men.

Rehydrate

Drink plenty of water before you go to bed and take a glass of water with you to sip if you wake in the night. A squeeze of fresh lemon juice in your water will lessen stomach acidity.

THE DAY AFTER

Drink plenty

Sip water to rehydrate yourself – aim for a glass every half an hour. Fresh fruit and vegetable juices are high in antioxidants and will help eliminate alcohol. Fizzy mineral water will reoxygenate your blood.

Supplement

Take a B-complex vitamin plus 1 g of vitamin C.

Avoid tea and coffee

Apart from being acidic and irritating the stomach, tea and coffee are diuretic and will make you lose any water you have left.

Eat well

Eat a healthy breakfast (see box opposite). Although you may feel like having a greasy fry-up, you'll regret it if you do – bacon, eggs and bread are all acid-forming, and will make your stomach churn even more. Eat foods that will not add to the body's toxic burden, such as brown rice, vegetables and nuts, throughout the day.

Mild exercise

Go for a long walk to purge the toxins.

Hydrotherapy

Have a relaxing bath before going to bed and try to get an early night.

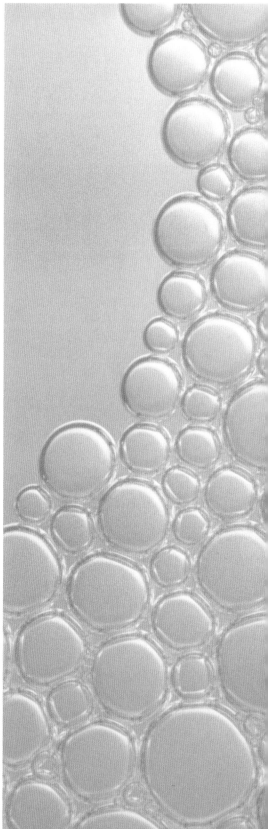

index